PRE-MENSTRUAL SYNDROME DIET AGAINST IT

ABOUT THE AUTHOR

Robert C.D. Wilson M.B. Ch.B. trained as a doctor in Aberdeen and after taking up posts in teaching and research in England and Canada he ran a general and preventive medical practice specialising in PMS in Vancouver. He now practices in London and has recently set up a preventive PMS clinic at the Marie Stopes Clinic as part of their Well Woman Service. He is married with a son and daughter.

PRE-MENSTRUAL SYNDROME DIET AGAINST IT

Robert C.D. Wilson M.B. Ch.B.

foulsham

London • New York • Toronto • Sydney

The author cannot assume any medical or legal responsibility for use of any information contained herein; this book discusses a wide range of situations that may not apply in individual cases.

foulsham
Yeovil Road, Slough, Berkshire SL1 4JH

ISBN 0–572–01524–0
© 1988 by R.C.D. Wilson M.B. Ch.B. Originally published in Canada by Fitzhenry and Whiteside under title of "Controlling Pre-Menstrual Syndrome". This Anglicized edition Copyright © 1989 W. Foulsham and Co. Ltd.

Printed in Great Britain by St Edmundsbury Press Ltd., Bury St Edmunds, Suffolk.

Dedication

To all women, and to those millions who now do suffer pain, discomfort, misery and worry before and at period time; and to young adolescents who will be tomorrow's women.

To be informed is to know, and to know is to go forward with understanding and without fear.

Acknowledgements

Without the direction of Professor Harry Keen of Guy's Hospital Medical School, who pointed me to the Dunn Institute of Nutrition in Cambridge, where Professor Philip James sparked my interest in nutrition, I would probably never have become so involved with the Pre-Menstrual Syndrome. To these two eminent clinicians and teachers, I express my gratitude.

To my many patients, male and female, I extend my thanks for all the support and encouragement they have offered me, as Pre-Menstrual Syndrome is a two-edged sword.
I am grateful to Christine West, who assisted me in researching material for inclusion in Chapter 1 — PMS: An Introduction

To Karen Kain, prima ballerina, who prepared the picture exercise routine for stress reduction and weight control and to the Milk Marketing Board of Ontario for the picture dialogue, my sincere thanks.

Finally to Maureen Wilson, my wife, Certificant of Cordon Bleu, who has compiled a series of Cooking for Health recipes, my gratitude for the low sodium and low sugar recipes in Appendices B and C. And again to Maureen, who typed and retyped the manuscript, showed patience and understanding always, my profound indebtedness.

Contents

Diagrams, Charts and Tables

Chapter 1

PMS: An Introduction

The purpose of this book is to explore the condition known as Pre-Menstrual Syndrome (PMS) in the light of modern research and to offer effective, pragmatic, up-to-date treatment for its control and prevention. More than 70 per cent of women I have treated now have their symptoms either completely controlled or controlled to such a degree that life for them is again bearable and they are able to function well.

In writing this book I have four clear objectives:

1. To *inform* about PMS. Lack of information or misinformation often causes worsening of a problem;
2. To *advise* on a treatment regime that has been shown to be helpful and effective;
3. To *encourage* all women suffering from PMS to believe that a medical-nutritional treatment approach can be very effective — hormones such as progesterone and other drugs need only be used in severe cases, and
4. To *present* this information in a format that will allow full understanding of this complicated problem, and to encourage discussion between you and your doctor of the information.

It is my belief that PMS is not a psychological illness. It is physical and is due to clear abnormalities of body chemistry, or metabolism. However, the symptoms of PMS can be divided into two main groups: psychological mood changes and physical changes.

In a normal ovulatory cycle a complicated interaction of hormones and chemicals takes place between different parts of the brain — the hypothalamus and the pituitary gland — and the uterus and ovaries. This interaction causes certain levels of hormones and body chemicals to be present in the tissues and bloodstream; these produce the low-intensity symptoms that most women recognize as heralding their menstruation — mood changes (such as depression, irritability, food cravings and feelings of reduced self-worth) and/or physical changes (such as breast tenderness, abdominal bloating, weight gain and backache). Such symptoms are really very mild PMS and are called *molimina*. They indicate an ovulatory cycle and are normal; if, however, these symptoms increase in intensity, then molimina become true PMS.

It is estimated that more than 40 per cent of women all over the world suffer from PMS in varying degrees, and although it frequently starts at menarche (onset of menstruation), PMS may not become a problem to many women until the age of 30. The increasing maturity of the hypothalamus in women over 30 years of age, along with a lack of exercise and an increase in body fat, are important links in the causes of PMS. The impact of stress and the association of fatty-acid-based hormones — prostaglandins — add further strands to the intricate web which is PMS. The onset of PMS may follow the taking of oral contraceptives, or may occur when these drugs are stopped. Operations such as hysterectomy, sterilization or even the insertion of an intrauterine contraceptive device (IUD) may cause the condition to occur. There would also seem to be a hereditary link. If a mother has the problem, then her daughters have approximately a 70 per cent chance of developing similar problems. It is interesting to note that adopted daughters tend to follow the same menstrual pattern as their natural mothers.

PMS has no preference for one race over another, although culture does appear to affect the type and severity of some of the symptoms. Breast symptoms are high in Japanese women, while Nigerians are affected more by headaches. American women appear to suffer more from backache than headache, and more from breast soreness than breast engorgement.

Nor does PMS affect one level of society; all may be touched by it. The pervasiveness of PMS in society generally, and the behaviour of many women whose lives are written in biographies, diaries, letters and chronicles, suggest that PMS may well have greatly influenced their daily functioning. Such is the impression created by Carolly Erickson in her book *Bloody Mary*, a life of Mary Tudor, and by Alison Plowden writing about Queen Elizabeth I in *Marriage with my Kingdom*.

Perhaps the most convincing are the 'Dear Child' letters written by Prince Albert to Queen Victoria at times when they had arguments. The letters reveal how cyclical the queen's temper was, and list the forms her uncontrolled behaviour took; she was also known to have screaming attacks, violent episodes during which she would throw things. As well, she suffered from severe post-partum depression.

Others who may have suffered from PMS include Pauline Bonaparte, sister of Napoleon, who is described as a volatile beauty who had to be treated on numerous occasions — and cyclically — for headaches, hysteria and bouts of temper, as well as for depression. Judy Garland suffered mood swings, depression, insomnia and compulsive eating; all of which worsened after the birth of her three children. She became dependent on medication, which she took to suppress her appetite. Maria Callas was well known for her temper outbursts, emotionalism, poor self-esteem and negative self-worth. She, too, suffered from binge eating. Documents show that her abnormal behaviour and attitude patterns took place in cycles each month. This may well fit the pattern of Pre-Menstrual Syndrome.

When Dr. Robert T. Frank of New York wrote on hormonal causes of pre-menstrual tension in 1931, his work was regarded as being without foundation. Time passed, and women continued to suffer the humiliation of being told that their complaints and problems of pre-menstruation had no foundation and were imaginary. In 1953 Dr. Raymond Greene, in association, with Dr. Katharina Dalton, published the first significant work on PMS in the *British Medical Journal*.

In 1980, 36-year-old Christine English killed her lover, running him down with her car. In 1981 Sandra Craddock, a 28-year-old barmaid from East London, fatally stabbed another barmaid. Both women were charged with murder; both their defence lawyers pleaded Pre-Menstrual Syndrome as part of their defence. In both cases Dr. Katharina Dalton gave evidence in their defence. After full medical evaluation, and on the advice of other physicians, the defendants were ordered by the court to receive treatment from Dr. Dalton. The evidence that Dr. Dalton gave, combined with each woman's improved pre-menstrual behaviour following treatment, convinced the court to impose lesser penalties. Sandra Craddock was released on probation, but was ordered to continue treatment with progesterone; the murder charge against her was reduced to manslaughter on the grounds of diminished responsibility. Christine English also had her murder charge reduced to manslaughter on the grounds of diminished responsibility; she was ordered by the court to receive treatment and was put on probation.

These are just two examples — albeit extreme cases — of the ravages that PMS can wreak upon human lives. It is a tragedy that it took such violence to bring PMS into focus and to give it the recognition by the medical profession that it deserves. Now that the existence of PMS as a medical disorder is acknowledged, it is equally important that its treatment should be effective, managed with consideration, and managed within the social context of a woman's life.

Chapter 2

Basics First: Inside Your Cycle

Puberty is the time of sexual awakening. It is the time of external evidence of a major internal chemical change. Some of the chemicals involved are called hormones. These complex chemical structures are released from the pituitary gland, situated in the brain. A part of the brain called the hypothalamus controls the amounts of hormones released from the pituitary gland. The two most relevant hormones are *FSH* — follicle stimulating hormone — and *LH* — luteinizing hormone. Collectively known as gonadotrophins, these are the nourishing hormones that stimulate the ovaries to produce *oestrogen* and cause ovulation.

At puberty it is mainly the hormone oestrogen that is flooding into the bloodstream, causing the early 'budding' of breast tissue and influencing the development of fat deposits, smoothing the body contours to produce the characteristic female outline. The growth of pubic and underarm hair begins; so also does sweat gland development. A young woman becomes interested in her body appearance and also in boys. Oestrogen also causes enlargement of the ovaries. From the size of a grape at puberty, over the next 12 to 24 months each ovary grows to become as large as a walnut. They are then ready for egg production.

Under the influence of FSH and LH from the pituitary gland, the first menstruation, known as the *menarche*, occurs. This represents a major change — the step from girlhood to womanhood, and with it the possibility of Pre-Menstrual Syndrome in some degree. The time of menarche varies, and seems to be influenced by factors such as race, genes, diet and socio-economic level. In certain New Guinea tribes the average age for menarche is 18 years, while in Cuba it is around 12.5 years. Mentally disabled girls, and those with Down's Syndrome, have a later menarche than girls with congenital abnormalities such as spina bifida. In Britain there has been a reduction in the age of menarche during the last century, from 17.5 years to approximately 14 years, due in most part, it is thought, to improved nutrition.

During the first year following menarche, usually only three or four episodes of menstruation — called periods — occur, with an average length of five to six days. As a girl progresses into her teens, the cycles usually shorten, and menstruation settles down to a two- or three-month pattern, with the bleeding phase lasting an average of five days. Male company, and male contacts, stimulate female menstrual hormones, and this in turn tends to regulate menstruation.

For simplicity in this discussion, the reproductive cycle lasts an average of 28 days, though in practice the length of the cycle can range from 20 to 36 days, due to the differing times in the month at which ovulation occurs. The first 14 days of the cycle are called the *follicular phase*, and the last 14 days, from ovulation to the onset of menstruation, are called the *luteal phase*. The duration of the menstrual flow may also change from month to month, lasting from two to eight days. Such a range is perfectly normal; so is the variable quantity of the menstrual flow.

Usually within two years of puberty, the process of ovulation begins. At birth the ovaries contain approximately 300,000 immature egg cells. No changes occur until menarche, when FSH causes these egg cells to mature, usually one at a time.

At the same time, other adjacent special cells produce the oestrogen hormone, which is released into the bloodstream and has a powerful effect on the inner lining of the uterus, called the *endometrium*, causing it to thicken and become rich in blood vessels. Meanwhile the growing, ripening egg cell has pushed its way to the surface of the ovary, where it produces a blister, or *follicle*. This ripening process takes approximately 14 days, and when it is complete the pituitary gland spills its luteinizing hormone (LH) into the blood stream. LH causes the ripened follicle to rupture and its egg cell floats free — the process known as *ovulation*.

At the burst follicle site LH causes different cells to accumulate, and these produce the second ovarian hormone, called *progesterone*. Progesterone causes the new tissue of the endometrium, which had been laid down under the direction of oestrogen during the follicular phase, to become softer and more spongelike, ready to receive a fertilized egg.

The walls of the vagina are kept moist by cells that produce mucus. During the follicular phase, oestrogen produced by the ovary causes this mucus to be thin, watery and clear, making easier the passage of any sperm towards the Fallopian tubes. During the luteal phase, after ovulation, the progesterone produced by the ruptured ovarian follicle (now called the *corpus luteum*) causes the vaginal mucus to thicken and become more tenacious; the mucus hinders further sperm from entering the Fallopian tubes. Progesterone also causes

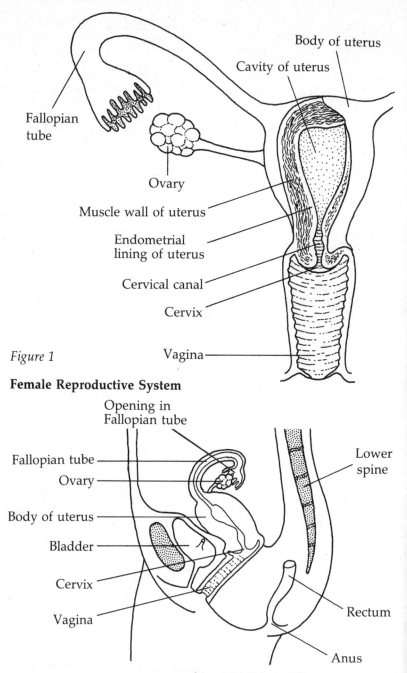

Body of uterus

Cavity of uterus

Fallopian
tube

Ovary

Muscle wall of uterus

Endometrial
lining of uterus

Cervical canal

Cervix

Figure 1

Vagina

Female Reproductive System

Opening in
Fallopian tube

Fallopian tube

Ovary

Body of uterus

Bladder

Cervix

Vagina

Lower
spine

Rectum

Anus

wavelike contractions of the tubes, assisting the egg in its six-and-a-half day voyage to the uterus.

If a sperm and egg unite, conception takes place, and the fertilized egg (*ovum*) embeds in the soft endometrial layer of the uterus. The delicate communication system that links the hypothalamus, pituitary, ovary and uterus is then activated, and quickly the progesterone blood level is increased, and maintained, to ensure adequate care and health of the endometrium of the uterus. The continuing progesterone production by the ovary is assured by the formation of a corpus luteal cyst at or near the site of the ovarian follicle. This progesterone production is then assisted greatly, after about the ninth week of pregnancy, by additional progesterone produced in the developing placenta. Recent research indicates that adequate levels of the hormone *prolactin* in the bloodstream are necessary for normal corpus luteal function and for further progesterone production to maintain a healthy pregnancy. Exactly how prolactin fits into the normal cycle is as yet unclear, but it is known that the hypothalamus has a regulatory function over its production and release by the pituitary gland.

Chart 1 **Hormone Changes During the Menstrual Cycle**

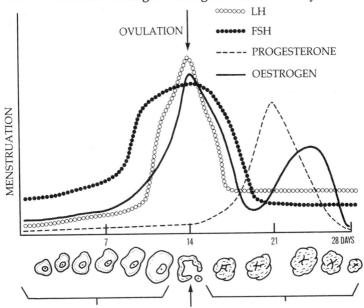

DEVELOPING FOLLICLE OVULATION CORPUS LUTEUM

15

Menstrual Cycle Hormone Paths

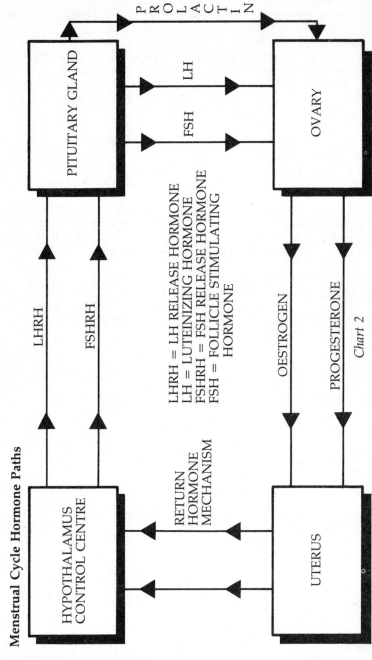

LHRH = LH RELEASE HORMONE
LH = LUTEINIZING HORMONE
FSHRH = FSH RELEASE HORMONE
FSH = FOLLICLE STIMULATING
        HORMONE

Chart 2

16

If conception does not take place, progesterone and oestrogen continue to be produced by the ovary until approximately the twenty-fourth day of the cycle. At this point the communication mechanism is again activated, with the hypothalamus reducing its releasing hormone to the pituitary, which in turn decreases its FSH and LH to the ovary. Consequently, during the last three days of the cycle there is a dramatic falling off of both oestrogen and progesterone. This leads to decreased blood flow to the uterus, which results in cell destruction, with shedding of the un-nourished inner uterine lining. The menstrual flow begins, removing the discarded, unwanted endometrium.

Menstruation is often accompanied by cramps. These are really contractions of the muscle wall of the uterus, squeezing the endometrium free and assisting in its expulsion. Recent intensive research has shown that the damaged endometrial cells release hormone-like substances called *prostaglandins*. These substances, like vitamins, have been given letter names; the prostaglandins that cause the uterus to contract or 'cramp' are of the E and F series. Prostaglandins are of immense importance in the overall balance mechanism of the body, and they may well hold a key role in the final control of PMS.

Chapter 3

PMS: Symptoms and Causes

Pre-Menstrual Syndrome is the cyclical repetition of symptoms, on or after ovulation, often increasing in severity up to the time of menstruation, followed by a complete absence of symptoms from the end of menstruation to ovulation. Because tension is probably the most common symptom complaint, the condition is sometimes referred to as Pre-Menstrual Tension, or PMT. However, the term *syndrome* is better, because it embraces multiple symptoms.

PMS symptoms can be divided into two groups, psychological (mood) changes and physical changes.

Table 1: Common PMS Symptoms

Psychological Changes Tension Depression Irritability Mood swings Feelings of losing control Altered sexual drive Hunger and food cravings, especially for sweet foods and chocolate Feelings of insecurity Reduced feelings of self-worth Outbursts of anger and hostility Suicidal thoughts and impulses
Physical Changes Headaches and migraine attacks Abdominal bloating and discomfort Sore breasts and breast fullness Lower back pain Weight gain Fatigue and loss of energy

Other conditions which I have found to be associated with, or aggravated by, the pre-menstruum are: varicose veins, acne, epilepsy, hypoglycaemia, alcohol excess, frequent urination, herpes breakout, asthma, allergies and pre-disposition to Candida (yeast) infections of the vagina, as well as infections of the eye and throat.

Symptoms often start abruptly, on or after the day of ovulation. Different symptoms may occur from one month to the next, and the severity of the symptoms may vary. A number of patients have told me how they may wake up one morning and feel "like a different person" — it is "as though a light had been switched off"; so rapid can the change be that being "one person one day and another the next" does indeed happen. Some patients encounter minor symptoms at ovulation time which subside, only to recur a few days later, then increase until menstruation begins, and then abate as rapidly as they began.

It is important to make clear here the difference between true PMS, spasmodic dysmenorrhoea and menstrual distress. Symptoms of true PMS begin at or shortly after ovulation and end at or shortly after menstruation begins, as in Type I or II in Chart 3. There is a complete absence of symptoms for at least seven to ten days after menstruation.

Spasmodic dysmenorrhoea is the occurrence at or just before the onset of menstruation of severe cramping pains in the lower abdomen, often radiating down the inner thigh area and frequently accompanied by vomiting and backache. Spasmodic dysmenorrhoea may be a part of *menstrual distress*, which is the occurrence of symptoms during any phase of the menstrual cycle (see Chart 4). These symptoms may come and go in a haphazard fashion throughout the cycle, but are most severe just before and during menstruation. If symptoms are present from menstruation to ovulation as in Type A, B or C, then true PMS is *not present*; causes other than PMS should be looked for. These other causes are detailed in Chapter 4 — Making the Diagnosis.

Many PMS symptoms are linked by common origin. For example, hostility, aggressive behaviour, panic attacks, epilepsy, headache, food cravings and increased appetite are due to *altered blood sugar levels*. Altered blood sugar levels and resulting reactive hypoglycaemia are very important and are discussed later in this chapter.

Bloatedness, breast tenderness, weight gain, body swelling (oedema) and backache are all due to *water retention*. The cause of water retention is uncertain, but a substance in the blood plasma called renin is raised in the luteal phase of the cycle, and causes an increase in levels of a substance called angiotensin II, stimulating thirst and altering the flow of water from cell to cell. Fatigue, tiredness, tension and depression are

Usual Timing of Symptoms in PMS

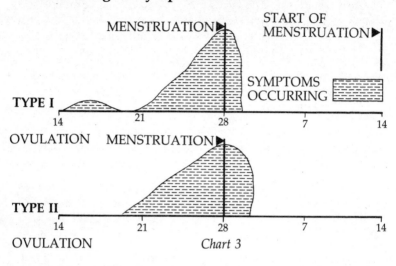

Chart 3

Frequent Symptoms Variation in Menstrual Distress

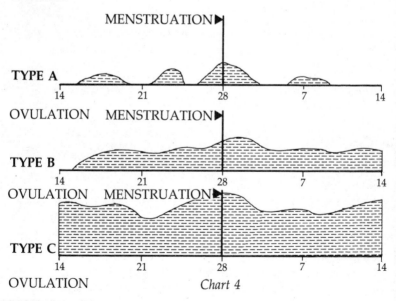

Chart 4

due to *sodium and potassium imbalance* (page 39).

Progesterone has a protective effect against infection and a reducing effect upon allergies. If a deficiency of progesterone is present during the luteal phase, then asthma, skin eruptions, acne and herpes are more likely to become troublesome.

An excessive sexual desire — increased libido — just before menstruation is often present in women suffering from PMS; in true depression, libido is reduced right through the cycle.

Researchers have found greater work absenteeism in the few days leading up to menstruation, during menstruation and at ovulation time. Hospital admissions increase significantly for women in their pre-menstrual phases, and about 50 per cent of all attempted and successful suicides by women occur during the pre-menstrual and menstrual phases.

There is unlikely to be one single cause for the multiplicity of PMS symptoms in any one patient at any one time. Poor nutrition, food additives such as monosodium glutamate (MSG) and tartrazine, convenience fast foods, caffeine and simple sugars can all cause or aggravate some of the symptoms of PMS. Stress in many forms can worsen PMS and the syndrome itself can cause stress in a marriage or relationship; thus the cycle of events feeds on itself.

It is now over 50 years since Dr. Robert Frank's article was written on Pre-Menstrual Tension, and over 30 years since Drs. Raymond Greene and Katharina Dalton published their joint paper "The Pre-Menstrual Syndrome", in the *British Medical Journal*. Since that time a great deal of research has taken place throughout the world into the reasons why some women exhibit symptoms of PMS and others do not.

The menstrual cycle is complex and can be influenced at any level by numerous hormone and nerve-centre actions. There exist several factors which, if defective or deficient in action, may produce PMS symptoms, the severity of which will depend upon the seriousness of the 'fault'. None of the following factors *cause* PMS individually, but they may contribute to the causes or influence the symptoms.

The HPO Factor

In the majority of women, menarche may herald the beginning of PMS; conversely, the end of the menopause signals the end of PMS. It is therefore logical to believe that the fine-tuning mechanism that is responsible for the body's delicate hormone balance–the hypothalamus-pituitary-ovary (HPO) nerve linkup–is faulty in some women.

In the luteal phase of the menstrual cycle there is a rising progesterone level; however, still present is a high blood level of oestrogen, in the form of oestradiol. Both progesterone and oestradiol are present in the blood plasma in two forms, the bound and the free; the bound form is attached to other proteins, while the free form is available and ready to be picked up or attached to receptor or target cells in different organs and areas of the body.

Recent research has produced evidence of lower plasma levels of progesterone in women with PMS. It is also known that progesterone, like prolactin, is not produced in an even flow during the luteal phase of the cycle, but rather in pulselike spurts. It may therefore be more accurate to measure the breakdown product of progesterone, which is pregnanediol, and which is excreted in the urine. Research confirms that there is reduced pregnanediol excretion by women diagnosed as having PMS. Therefore, progesterone in such women is likely to be deficient.

If the HPO nerve linkup is malfunctioning, then the free oestradiol-progesterone balance is upset, and this in turn may reduce the calming effect on tissues and organs which progesterone is known to produce. For example, it reduces brain activity, with resulting lessening of convulsions, thereby also reducing the possibility of epilepsy pre-menstrually. In a similar way, if this fine balance is altered, the calming effect can break or modify the reactive hypoglycaemic cycle and its accompanying food craving by reducing the insulin influence from the pancreas.

Asthma and certain body infections may be reduced, because of the smoother action of the hormone balance upon the immune system.

The Endorphin Factor

Specific peptides — α-melanocyte stimulating hormone (α-MSH) and β-endorphin — produced by a specific part of the hypothalamus — may be responsible for the occurrence of PMS in susceptible women, or in those where the α-MSH or β-endorphin are produced in excess. These peptide substances may trigger the pituitary to produce prolactin, and they also greatly influence prostaglandin activity, as well as possibly affecting the production of vasopressin — a pituitary hormone that regulates blood pressure — thereby producing headaches and tension.

The Prolactin Factor

The pituitary hormone prolactin occurs in both sexes, but at puberty increases more in females. Its production is controlled by the hypothalamus, by a substance thought to be dopamine, which assists and transmits electrical nerve impulses. During the menstrual cycle, prolactin is released into the bloodstream in a pulsatile manner. Stress, surgical operations and breast manipulation can all cause an increase in prolactin production. Too much prolactin can reduce the amount of progesterone released in the luteal phase of the cycle, thereby worsening some PMS symptoms. A prolactin excess – also caused by a lack of prostaglandin E1 (below) – has a direct effect on the breasts, causing swelling, pain and tenderness.

The Prostaglandin Factor

Prostaglandins, hormone-like substances produced from fatty acids, are present in most body cells. They are identified, like vitamins, by code letter and number, such as $E1$, $E2$, $F1$, $F2$. They alter the body chemistry and their influence is widespread, especially upon smooth-muscle contractions in areas such as the heart, intestines, blood vessels and uterus.

Prostaglandins may act alone or in concert. Often it is the quantitative relationship of one to the other that determines how well or how badly an organ is functioning. For instance, because prostaglandins can regulate the size of blood vessels, they can increase or reduce sodium and water excretion from the kidneys. This in turn can influence blood pressure and cause headaches. Menstrual cramps are a result of normal uterine contractions. In spasmodic dysmenorrhoea, these cramps are abnormal, giving rise to debilitating pain, and often a sufferer has to go to bed. It has been found that prostaglandin $F2$ and $E2$ are responsible for this abnormality, and that certain anti-prostaglandin drugs, which block the prostaglandin action, can be helpful. Two available Prostaglandin inhibitor drugs include Mefenamic acid and Naproxen.

Prostaglandins are of vital importance to total body function; but so too is progesterone, and so too is the HPO nerve linkup. If there is a defect in the overall HPO relationship, then symptoms of illness will occur. PMS is an example of this. To maintain this delicate balance, it is necessary to ensure adequate production of prostaglandins. The building blocks of prostaglandins are *essential fatty acids*. The body cannot manufacture these, and so they have to be taken in through the diet in the same way as minerals, vitamins and essential amino acids. If the intake of essential fatty acids is deficient, then prostaglandin production will fall, with resulting illness such as skin problems, allergic conditions and hormone imbalance.

Essential fatty acids primarily have vegetable origins. Some of the better known are palmitic, stearic, oleic and *linoleic*. It is *linoleic acid* (LA), that the body requires to manufacture several of the prostaglandins, especially the E1 series. LA is therefore helpful in reducing the symptoms of PMS. The main food source of essential fatty acids is polyunsaturated vegetable oil such as sunflower oil, safflower oil and corn oil. These contain respectively approximately 58 per cent, 73 per cent and 58 per cent of LA in the beneficial *cis* form. (All fatty acids contain hydrocarbon chains, which vary in the number of carbon atoms they contain. The carbon atoms may be joined by single or double bonds. If there exist two similar atom groupings on the same side of the double bond, then a *cis* configuration of the fatty acid molecule is said to exist.)

Polyunsaturated refers to the number of double bonds in the hydrocarbon chemical structure. Treatment with hydrogen gas, a process called hydrogenation, converts liquid oil into a firmer, semi-solid and spreadable substance — such as margarine. Hydrogenation, however, transforms the fatty acids in the oil to a less beneficial *trans* form and reduces the number of double bonds in its molecule. Much of the LA is destroyed and, therefore, is not available for prostaglandin manufacture. It is very important that margarine packages clearly state how much cis-LA they contain. It is my opinion that if there is not a statutory minimum percentage, as in the case of special margarines with a minimum of *trans* fatty acids that make a claim to be high in polyunsaturates, then they are not a suitable source of natural LA.

LA occurs in the *cis* form, in its natural state, and the body must convert it to prostaglandin E1 in a complicated chain of events. This conversion process is shown in Chart 5, with the nutritional factors required for each stage. The process may be hindered by body illness such as heart disease, elevated cholesterol levels, excess alcohol ingestion, diabetes mellitus, and low vitamin intake as well as by an excess intake of animal fats and processed vegetable oils such as block margarine. These cholesterol-rich animal fats and hydrogenated, processed vegetable oils compete for the cis-LA available and may cause a reduction in the formation of gamma-linolenic acid (GLA).

The first stage in the conversion of LA to prostaglandin E1 produces GLA. If natural sources of LA are not readily

Prostaglandin *E1* Formation from *Linoleic* Acid

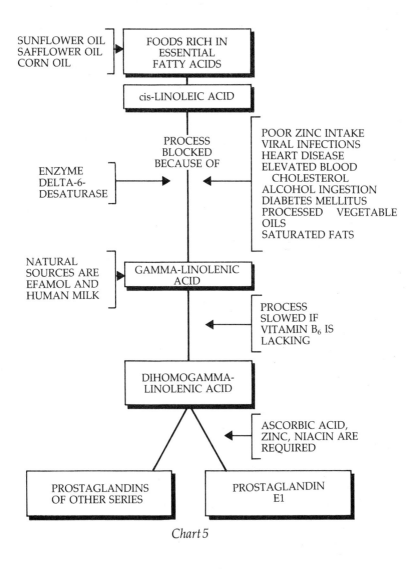

Chart 5

available, or if increased ingestion of GLA is considered advisable in PMS treatment, then the product Efamol can be used. (GLA, available as Efamol in capsule form, is discussed in Chapter 5 — Treatment of PMS.) Human breast milk, though impractical for adult consumption, is also a rich source of GLA. Considerable loss and drain of GLA occurs from the mother's body when she breast feeds, and this may be one reason why successive pregnancies increase the incidence and risk of post-partum depression and PMS.

Both Dr. Michael Brush in England and Dr. David Horrobin in Canada have contributed greatly in their individual research to the understanding of LA and its relationship to PMS.

The Hypoglycaemia Factor

During the pre-menstrual phase the body's ability to cope correctly with carbohydrate foods — especially simple sugars — is significantly altered. The body has two important mechanisms for dealing with blood sugar — one in the pancreas and the other in the adrenal glands.

The pancreas produces insulin, and the adrenal glands adrenalin. Insulin lowers blood sugar. Adrenalin raises it. The eating of too much simple carbohydrate — often in the form of sweet foods (food cravings) — raises the blood glucose level until the pancreas is forced, through its sensitive islet cells, to trigger the insulin mechanism. This reduces the blood sugar. In sufferers from PMS the triggering mechanism in the adrenal glands is more sensitive to the lowered blood sugar, and therefore produces more adrenalin sooner; this causes an adrenalin rush, with consequent explosive temper, panic attacks, fainting, epileptic seizures, and migraine onset. The longer one goes without food, the worse the situation can become. These episodes of reactive hypoglycaemia also produce the ravenous appetite and food cravings typical in some women as the time of menstruation approaches. Reactive hypoglycaemia must not be confused with true hypoglycaemia, which usually has a different cause and is often due to disease within the pancreas itself. Reactive hypoglycaemia, though not the cause of PMS, occurs in many women who do have PMS symptoms, and is considered an influencing factor in producing some of the symptoms.

Simple carbohydrates in the form of sugar and highly refined processed foods are the biggest villains. These are the foods that most readily trigger the oversensitive mechanism in the adrenal glands. By alteration of diet, the above symptoms can be greatly reduced. The importance of diet in the overall control of PMS symptoms cannot be overemphasized.

The Immune Factor

The body has a defence system against attack from foreign irritants and infections, the so-called antigens. This system depends upon a healthy lymph system, at the core of which are the white cells, especially the macrophages and lymphocytes, in the form of B and T cells. Macrophages attack the antigens and alter them for easier assault by assisting cells called lymphocytes. Macrophages also release prostaglandins, which play a vital role in the other body defence mechanism, inflammation. Lymphocytes, when triggered to act in defence, may, if healthy, produce certain immunoglobulins from their B cells. There are four main groups of immunoglobulins: IgA, IgM, IgG and IgE.

IgA provides protection in areas of the body where mucous membranes are involved. A deficiency of IgA is associated with a tendency to develop infections, especially of the intestine. IgE is the immunoglobulin involved in such conditions as asthma, drug reactions, rhinitis, allergic conjunctivitis, cow's milk allergy in infants, and food allergies with accompanying skin reactions such as hives, eczema and 'nettle rash'.

A deficiency of prostaglandins, including the D2 series, can lead to a breakdown in the immune system. This explains why conditions such as asthma, rhinitis and repeated infections of the mouth and vagina (*Candida albicans*) may occur before menstruation.

Research has shown that any imbalance of prostaglandins in the body can lead to skin problems such as eczema, or other conditions such as asthma, hay-fever or sinusitis in individuals who show a higher susceptibility to such conditions because of their overreaction to antigens in the environment. Such persons are called *atopic*. This type of overreaction is sometimes genetic. I have observed that a high proportion of women with PMS also have allergy problems or had eczema or asthma when a child; these conditions are also quite common in their families.

Recently pre-menstrual migraine has also been linked to prostaglandin imbalance. This again indicates the close relationship between prostaglandins and progesterone and the immune system. Some pre-menstrual migraine headaches respond dramatically to the administration of progesterone or prostaglandin inhibitor drugs.

Mono-amine Oxidase (MAO) Factor

Recent research has shown the presence in the brain and in the blood of an enzyme called mono-amine oxidase. MAO breaks down, through biochemical processes, some amine substances called neurotransmitters such as dopamine, serotonin and noradrenaline. By preventing neurotransmitters from becoming too strong, MAO produces a calming effect. On the other hand, too little MAO allows greater brain activity, and therefore more irritability and mood changes.

Mono-amines are necessary for the body's normal function. Many common foods contain healthy levels of amines (see Table 2), and the body can often handle these outside sources, usually in the form of tyramine, very well. However, in certain cases there is a hereditary deficiency of MAO, and the breakdown of mono-amines fails to take place as it should. The resulting rise in body amines can aggravate or even cause PMS symptoms such as headaches and alterations to mood and even affect the menstrual cycle. In treating severe PMS the removal of amine-rich foods from the diet can be very helpful.

Table 2

Foods High in Amines

Foods	Amines
Bananas	Serotonin, dopamine, tyramine, noradrenaline
Raisins	Mono-amines
Cheese	Tyramine
Avocado	Tyramine, dopamine
All liver	Tyramine
Herring, kippers, anchovies	Tyramine
Mushrooms	Tyramine
Broad beans	Dopamine
Sour cream	Tyramine
Soy and Worcestershire sauce	Tyramine
Oranges and tangerines	Tyramine, synephrine
Tomatoes	Tryptamine, serotonin

Chapter 4

Making the Diagnosis

Some doctors still feel that PMS does not exist, or that if it does, it is in the mind of the distraught woman, and a cure consists of firm words such as, "You had better snap out of it, otherwise you may lose your husband, your job or both". Younger women may be less willing to discuss their fears and symptoms and may become withdrawn and frightened. It is not unusual for a husband, boyfriend or close relative to first notice that a 'different person' exists at a certain time each month. Prodding from a friend or relative is what often encourages the sufferer to seek help.

This is where PMS becomes one of personal involvement for you. You understand your menstrual cycle. You realize that you are not alone in having certain symptoms during the menstrual cycle — over 40 per cent of all women do — and you also know that such symptoms can vary in type and severity. What you now wish to know is whether your symptoms are those of PMS.

Your Doctor

As I have said, not all doctors are in sympathy with PMS, and indeed there are those who do not understand it. Selecting, then, your professional advisor is very important. You will already know, perhaps, your family physician's approach to medical problems. You will know if your physician is easy to talk to and whether you feel comfortable discussing intimate and personal problems with him or her. If you question this, speak to some of your friends; get their advice as to whom they consult. If you have a good friend with PMS, find out from her who her doctor is; after all, improvement in a friend suffering from PMS is a strong recommendation of the physician who is giving her advice and assistance.

During the last ten years or so many doctors have assumed a more humanistic, health-oriented, preventive approach to patient care, taking in diet, exercise, and lifestyle. I feel that this holistic approach, where the entire picture of illness is considered in the context of a patient's family, job, lifestyle, stress factors and dietary-nutritional background, is the only way in which PMS can successfully be diagnosed and treated.

29

The First Visit — History Taking

The first contact a patient usually has in a doctor's surgery is with the receptionist. She is often a very good indicator of how comfortable your initial visit there may be. Does she rush you on the telephone, or does she give you the impression that you are being listened to? Is she warm, friendly and helpful? Is she able to tell you that the doctor does treat PMS and has an interest in the problem?

When a patient first comes to see me wondering if she has PMS, or with symptoms she does not understand, I will discuss with her her life in general, the type of work she is engaged in and her position in the family. She then becomes more relaxed, and more communicative. A patient must always be made to feel that a doctor has time for her. Because tension, anxiety and irritability often play an important role in the way a woman with PMS feels, it is understandable that she may be more nervous and upset at the time of her first doctor's appointment. She should therefore try to schedule her first appointment at a time when her cycle is most comfortable for her. (Personally, however, I feel it advantageous to have first-visit appointments with women suspected of having PMS during their pre-menstrual phase, for symptoms are then often at or near their height and are more vivid: nervousness, facial swelling or puffiness and a less tolerant attitude towards others may be quite evident to one who is looking for them.)

I schedule the first visit for approximately one hour. This visit is very important to both of us. You, at last, have someone to talk to, who will listen to what you have to say. At last someone reassures you that the symptoms you are experiencing are real. You *do* have them. They are not imaginary. You are then asked questions about your symptoms, and your answers are recorded. The severity of your symptoms is graded on a scale from 1 to 5. The time of the month when the symptoms occur is noted, with particular attention to when the menstrual period begins and ends. Depression symptoms in particular must be evaluated with care to exclude serious forms of depression or a manic depressive illness.

Listed below is an example of typical symptoms, followed by the severity coding that the patient feels is appropriate. A similar list can easily be made up by yourself and taken with you on the first visit to your doctor.

Depression .... ++ (2)   Name _____
Irritability .... +++ (3)
Tension .... +++ (3)   Birthdate_____
Tiredness .... +++ (3)
Weight gain .... ++ (2)
Bloated feeling .... ++ (2)
Backache .... + (1)
Lack of concentration .... ++ (2)
Food cravings .... +++ (3)

Questions are then asked in the following categories (you may wish to complete these questions before you see your doctor):

Personal History Questionnaire

1. **Menstrual History and Contraception**

   a) When did your periods begin? _____
   b) Length of cycle? _____
   c) Length of bleeding phase? _____
   d) Do you have pain at menstruation? _____
   e) Do you have pain at other times in the menstrual cycle? If so, discuss. _____ _____
   f) Have you ever used birth control pills? _____
   g) Have you ever had an intrauterine contraceptive device? _____

2. **Past and Present Medical-Surgical History**

   a) What surgical operations have you had? _____
   b) List your past illnesses. _____ _____
   c) Did any require hospitalization? _____ _____
   d) Do you have heart problems (high blood pressure, palpitations, etc.)? _____ _____
   e) Do you have lung problems (asthma, chronic cough, infections)? _____
   f) Do you have gastrointestinal problems (pain, bloating, constipation)? _____

3. **Personal History and Allergies**

   a) Have you ever been pregnant? _____
   b) Have you had a miscarriage or an abortion? _____

c) Do you have, or have you had, vaginal infections? ___

d) Do they occur at a particular time in your menstrual cycle? _____

e) Do your breasts become lumpy or painful before your period? _____

f) Have you ever taken antibiotics? What for, and what kind? _____

g) Have you any known allergies? _____

h) Do you react to any medications? _____

i) Are you sensitive to any vapours, perfumes, cleaning products, etc.? _____

j) Do any foods cause you problems? What are they? ___

k) Has your weight changed in the last 6 months? _____

l) Do you have headaches? How frequently and how severe? _____

m) Do you suffer from depression? All the time or just before your period? _____

n) Do you have anxiety? How severe? All the time or just before your period? _____

o) Do you have crying spells, lack of concentration, panic attacks or feel you are losing control? When in the cycle do you note these changes? _____

p) Do you take caffeine in any form — coffee, tea, cola drinks, chocolate? _____

q) Do you smoke cigarettes? How many per day? _____

r) Do you take, or have you taken, drugs? What kind?

s) Do you drink alcohol? How much and how often? ___

4. Family History

a) How many sisters have you? How old are they? _____

b) How is the health of your father and mother? _____

c) Have any female relatives been known to suffer from PMS? _____

d) Is there a family history of diabetes mellitus or depression?

5. **Exercise, Relaxation and Food-Monitoring**

Questions are asked of you concerning the type of exercise you do daily, as well as your forms of relaxation. The Food-Monitoring Chart, with spaces for recording exercises, relaxation and drugs/vitamins consumed each day (see Chart 6) is explained to you. You are given seven charts for consecutive days and are requested to bring them completed to your next appointment.

6. **Stress**

(Stress is discussed in Chapter 5 — Treatment of PMS.)

Example of a Typical Month Charting PMS Symptoms

You are also given a Menstrual Chart for Recording Symptoms (see Chart 7). Using codes, mark on the chart the symptoms you experience and rate their severity. For example: D = depression, H = headache; 1 = mild, 3 = moderate, 5 = severe. Complete this over a two-month time span *at least*. The completed chart (see Chart 8 for an example) shows your doctor when your symptoms begin and end in relation to your menstrual period and how severe your symptoms are; most importantly, it tells your doctor if your symptoms are cyclical — if they occur regularly month after month.

When your questionnaire and charts are completed, you and your doctor can review your history and chart findings. This could save two or three months' waiting and evaluation time, and treatment of symptoms can begin much sooner.

The Second Visit — Physical Examination

The second visit takes place seven to ten days after your first visit, and you should schedule this appointment during a time when you are not menstruating. I find I require another complete hour for this evaluation phase.

First, the history taken at the last visit is reviewed; you are asked if you have any further comments to make or items to add for completeness. You are asked if you have started the menstrual charting, and you hand in your Food-Monitoring Chart. This will be reviewed at the next appointment.

Daily Food-Monitoring Chart

TIME	FOOD EATEN	QUANTITY	MOOD	EXERCISE	RELAXATION	DRUGS & VITAMINS
BREAK-FAST						
MID-MORNING						
LUNCH						
AFTER-NOON						
DINNER						
EVENING						

Chart 6

Menstrual Chart for Recording Symptoms

DAYS OF THE MONTH

MONTH	1 2 3 4 5 6 7 8 9 10 11 12 13 14 15 16 17 18 19 20 21 22 23 24 25 26 27 28 29 30 31

MONTH	1 2 3 4 5 6 7 8 9 10 11 12 13 14 15 16 17 18 19 20 21 22 23 24 25 26 27 28 29 30 31

MONTH	1 2 3 4 5 6 7 8 9 10 11 12 13 14 15 16 17 18 19 20 21 22 23 24 25 26 27 28 29 30 31

D—DEPRESSION
I—IRRITABILITY
T—TIREDNESS
H—HEADACHE
TS—TENSION

B—BREAST DISCOMFORT
A—ABDOMEN BLOATING
LC—LACK OF COMMUNICATION (WITHDRAWN)

S—SWELLINGS
C—CLUMSINESS
WG—WEIGHT GAIN

FC—FOOD CRAVING
N—NAUSEA
AS—ASTHMA
PP—PAIN
M—MENSTRUATION

SEVERITY CODE

1+ ⟶ 5+
MILD   SEVERE

Chart 7

35

Example of a Typical Menstrual Chart

DAYS OF THE MONTH

1	2	3	4	5	6	7	8	9	10	11	12	13	14	15	16	17	18	19	20	21	22	23	24	25	26	27	28	29	30	31
						TS1	TS1	TS1	TS1	TS1	TS1	TS2	TS2	TS3	TS3	TS3	TS3	TS3	TS3	M	M	M	M	M						
						T1	T1	T1	T1	T1	T1	T1	T1	T2	T2	T2	T2	T2	T2											
						D1	D1	D1	D1	D1	D1	D1	D2	D2	D3	D2	D2	D3	O3											
												WG1	WG1	WG1	WG1	WG1	WG1													
							LC1	LC1	LC1	LC1	LC1	LC1	LC1	LC1	LC2	LC2	LC2	LC2	FC2											
													WG1	WG1	FC2	FC2	FC3	FC3	LC2											
																B2	B2	B2	B2											
																WG1	WG1	WG1.2	FC2											

MONTH _____ July _____

SEVERITY CODE

1+ MILD ——→ 5+ SEVERE

D—DEPRESSION
I—IRRITABILITY
T—TIREDNESS
H—HEADACHE
TS—TENSION
B—BREAST DISCOMFORT
A—ABDOMEN BLOATING
LC—LACK OF COMMUNICATION (WITHDRAWN)
S—SWELLINGS
C—CLUMSINESS
WG—WEIGHT GAIN
FC—FOOD CRAVING
N—NAUSEA
AS—ASTHMA
PP—PAIN
M—MENSTRUATION

Chart 8

The complete examination should include:
1. Measurement of blood pressure, weight and height.
2. Breast examination for lumps and breast milk production if any.
3. Inspection and palpation for thyroid disease.
4. Internal pelvic examination, to rule out pelvic disease such as endometriosis or infection. Constipation may also be detected with pain over the rectum.
5. Inspection of the skin, eyes and nasal mucosa for allergy or evidence of infection.
6. Inspection for excessive hair growth on the skin, especially on the face, abdomen or buttocks which may indicate hormone imbalance.

Certain laboratory and diagnostic tests should be done to rule out any existing or potential problems that may account for some of your symptoms. I do the following routinely; your own doctor may wish to consider them:
1. A complete blood count.
2. Thyroid screen.
3. Blood screen evaluation, which includes blood sugar, blood fats (cholesterol, triglycerides), sodium and potassium levels.
4. Protein evaluation.
5. Calcium.
6. Urine test.
7. Smear test.
8. If vaginal discharge or irritation is a complaint, a vaginal swab should be taken to detect any infection such as *Candida albicans* (yeast).
9. In cases of troublesome or severe headaches, I would consider taking a prolactin blood level on two consecutive days. This should be done if there is any abnormal discharge from the nipple.
10. At the discretion of your doctor, other hormone evaluations such as LH, FSH and Testosterone including levels of SHBG (a sex hormone binding agent), may be required.

The Third Visit

Approximately one hour is required for this important evaluation.

Your Food-Monitoring Chart (and the stress questionnaires discussed in Chapter 5 — The Treatment of PMS) are reviewed, and recommendations are made based on what they show. Diet, stress, exercise, relaxation and drugs/vitamins can greatly influence PMS, for it is not a single condition but a syndrome that involves the whole body. As well, your first month's Menstrual Chart for Recording PMS is reviewed. This is very helpful to your doctor because it indicates the type of menstrual pattern you have. You are both able to see quickly which symptoms are the most troublesome and when they occur.

Your doctor is now able to decide into which of the three menstrual patterns your symptoms fit, according to the timing of symptoms.

1. *Spasmodic dysmenorrhoea* — symptoms begin a few hours before menstruation only. The symptoms are usually a triad of pain, backache and vomiting, and are confined to menstruation only.
2. *Menstrual distress* — symptoms come and go in a haphazard fashion throughout the entire cycle, but are most severe just before and during menstruation. ·
3. *Pre-Menstrual Syndrome* — symptoms occur in the latter half of the cycle, with complete absence of symptoms for at least seven to ten days after menstruation.

The occurrence at a time *other than pre-menstrually* (from ovulation to the onset of menstruation) of such symptoms as depression, tiredness, headaches or migraine, asthma and food cravings, as well as pelvic pain or breast discharge, warrants careful and full evaluation. The presence of these symptoms at that time may indicate underlying disease.

Depression may be endogenous — without an obvious external cause. Persistent anxiety may indicate a neurosis. Psychiatric opinion and care may be required. Prolonged tiredness or weakness may indicate an underactive thyroid gland or lack of serum potassium due to inappropriate diuretic usage. Migraine or other headaches may be due to underlying allergy problems or to low blood sugar levels. Asthma attacks may have their cause in food or inhalant sensitivity or even in aspirin ingestion. Pelvic pain may be a symptom of endometriosis, a pelvic inflammatory disease, ovarian conditions or even chronic constipation. Breast discharge may be due to excessive prolactin production caused by a pituitary gland abnormality.

Obviously, very careful evaluation through history taking, menstrual-symptom charting, physical examination and laboratory tests are needed to determine accurately if either true PMS or menstrual distress is present. Stress, certain lifestyle habits (such as excessive drinking, smoking, lack of exercise, and eating too much sugar and refined foods) and chronic disease such as rheumatoid arthritis and cardiac problems can aggravate the symptoms of true PMS, but they can also greatly affect — and even cause — some of the symptoms of menstrual distress. It is not unusual for both conditions to co-exist; if this is the case, the symptoms of true PMS may be made worse by the existence of an underlying disease or malfunction that is causing the menstrual distress. It is very important, therefore, to correctly diagnose the causes of menstrual distress symptoms in order to begin effective treatment and to avoid confusion with Pre-Menstrual Syndrome.

The suspected diagnosis is then made and is confirmed after a review of your *second* monthly chart. Although your PMS symptoms may vary somewhat from month to month, generally each woman has six to eight dominant symptoms and several minor symptoms. Symptoms can often be grouped together because they may share a common cause (see Table 3).

Common Symptoms and Their Causes

Symptoms	Probable Causes
Headaches Aggression Fainting Lack of concentration Panic attacks Food cravings	Alteration in blood sugar levels
Weight gain Bloated feelings Breast tenderness Backache	Fluid retention
Lethargy Muscle weakness Irritability Tension	Imbalance of body electrolytes such as potassium and sodium
Migraine Asthma Herpes outbreak Other infection	Alteration in the body defence and immune system

Table 3

Timing of Symptoms in the Three Menstrual Patterns

DAYS OF THE MONTH

	1	2	3	4	5	6	7	8	9	10	11	12	13	14	15	16	17	18	19	20	21	22	23	24	25	26	27	28	29	30	31
PRE-MENSTRUAL SYNDROME															X	X	X	X	X	X	X	X	X	X	M	M	M	M			
MENSTRUAL DISTRESS									X	X						X	X	X					X	X	M	M	M	M	X		X
SPASMODIC DYSMENORRHOE.																								X	M X	M X	M	M			

X = DAYS ON WHICH SYMPTOMS OCCUR

M = DAYS ON WHICH MENSTRUATION OCCURS

Chart 9

40

It is not possible to place you in a single category for PMS, because different symptoms can occur from month to month, and because there are very different causes of those symptoms. It is possible, however, to know if your symptoms overall are mild, moderate or severe. This is done by assessing how you feel in the pre-menstrual and menstrual phases, and by linking this to your menstrual charting and the symptom severity code. You should, for example, be able to identify yourself with one of the three groups below:

Mild PMS Symptoms: I can function well without interruption of job, home life or marriage.
Moderate PMS Symptoms: I feel each month that something happens to me. I am like a different person, and I find coping with my work, friends and marriage is difficult. Relationships are suffering.
Severe PMS Symptoms: I feel I cannot go on like this, I am just not functioning normally. I am very depressed. I sometimes panic and become violent. I am afraid I may do something terrible.

Tell your doctor about your feelings and your fears. It is only through good communication, and careful evaluation of your symptoms, that the appropriate treatment for you can begin.

Chapter 5

The Treatment of PMS

Part I: Mild and Moderate PMS

After careful evaluation, the diagnosis has been made; you *do suffer* from PMS.

I have found that by employing a ten-point key regime there can be as much as 75 per cent improvement in the symptoms of mild and moderate PMS. The regime incorporates changes to diet and lifestyle.

Table 4

The Ten-Point Key Regime

1. Eliminate caffeine.
2. Reduce salt (sodium) intake.
3. Reduce simple carbohydrate intake and increase complex carbohydrate intake.
4. Increase dietary fibre.
5. Achieve adequate protein intake.
6. Eat regularly, and on time.
7. Eat snacks of complex carbohydrate or protein between meals.
8. Add linoleic acid or gamma-linolenic acid to diet.
9. Add necessary nutrients to diet (B-complex, vitamin B_6, vitamin C, folic acid, calcium, magnesium and zinc.)
10. Change lifestyle: reduce alcohol consumption.
    Stop smoking.
    Stop oral contraceptives.
    Manage stress through exercise and relaxation.

1. Eliminate caffeine

Although caffeine is a stimulant, it leads to short spurts of energy followed by bouts of tiredness and fatigue. Caffeine increases irritability and anxiety and causes mood swings. Because it increases blood flow, caffeine interferes with the absorption of B vitamins and may have a similar effect on iron, calcium and magnesium. Caffeine is usually consumed in the form of beverages such as coffee, tea and cola drinks; cocoa and some forms of chocolate also contain it. Coffee, percolated or instant, contains about three times more caffeine per six-ounce cup than tea. Most cola drinks contain in a twelve-ounce serving more caffeine than a six-ounce cup of tea brewed for three minutes. Many over-the-counter drugs such as those sold to relieve headache, or indeed menstrual pain and discomfort, contain caffeine. It is important to read the label before buying such drugs.

Caffeine should be avoided as much as possible. Good substitute beverages are weak tea, herb teas, water-processed decaffeinated coffee (Swiss process) and grain-based coffee substitutes. Ordinary decaffeinated coffee still contains some caffeine and, because of the chemical process involved in its preparation, may contain potential carcinogens.

2. Reduce salt (sodium) intake

Sodium is an essential nutrient that has important roles to play in the normal functioning of the body. These include maintaining blood volume and maintaining the required pressure within the body cells. An adequate daily sodium intake is thought to be around 3 g as common salt (sodium chloride, or NaCl).

Salt and high sodium foods increase fluid retention, bloating and breast tenderness. Sufferers of PMS should restrict their sodium intake to around 2 g of sodium chloride daily during the last two weeks of their menstrual cycle. Those living in hot climates or following a regimen of strenuous exercise may require more sodium. Your physician will be able to advise you on sodium intake depending upon your needs. Remember that sodium occurs in many forms. Common salt has the following conversion ratio: 1 g of salt is equivalent to 400 mg of sodium.

Before buying foods, read the labels and try to use products with as low a salt content as possible, especially during the *last half of your menstrual cycle*. Remember that sodium on the label may be shown as Na — the chemical name abbreviation. Wash all frozen, canned and smoked seafood well in cold water, wash cottage cheese in a fine-mesh sieve, and do not add salt to your food. Convenience foods and food from fast-food outlets usually have a high sodium content. Certain additives and preservatives such as monosodium glutamate (MSG) and sodium nitrite are present in a great many foods. Many baked goods contain baking powder — sodium bicarbonate — and many antacids contain sodium in large quantities.

Low and moderate sodium recipes are included in Appendices B and C to help you control your sodium intake.

High Sodium Foods and Alternatives

Food	Low Sodium Alternatives
Bacon, ham, salami, corned beef, frankfurters, sausages	Fresh meat and poultry
Frozen fish fillets, canned or smoked fish including sardines, salmon and herring	Fresh fish such as cod, mackerel, salmon, sole, trout, tuna — packed in water; low sodium canned vegetables and soups
All shellfish, shrimp, prawns and crab	
All cheeses	Low sodium cheeses; cottage cheese (unsalted or washed) Eggs
Peanut butter	Low sodium peanut butter
Salted butter	Unsalted butter
Commercial mayonnaise	Low salt mayonnaise
Salted nuts and dried fruit	Unsalted nuts
Baked goods	Baked goods containing sodium-free baking powder (potassium bicarbonate)
Mineral water with high sodium content	Low salt mineral water (e.g., Perrier)
Ketchup, etc.	Potassium-based salt substitute

Flavouring Aids

Barbecue sauce	Basil, chives, dill, fennel, garlic, mace, mint, nutmeg, oregano, rosemary, sage, sorrel, thyme, turmeric
Bouillon cubes	Fresh onion, shallot
Ketchup	Miso, tamari and soy sauce (¼ tsp. only has the seasoning power of 1 tsp. salt)
Celery salt, garlic salt, onion salt	Fresh onion, shallot, fresh and dried herbs
Cyclamates (artificial sweetness)	
Meat extracts and tenderizers	
Prepared mustard	
Pickles & Relishes	
Worcestershire sauce	

Table 5

3. Reduce simple carbohydrate intake and increase complex carbohydrate intake

Carbohydrates are the body's source of energy. Simple carbohydrates are composed of sugars and are usually sweet to the taste. They take the form of glucose, fructose, sucrose, lactose and maltose, to name a few. Simple carbohydrates are rapidly and easily digested by the enzymes in the saliva and bowel. They flood the blood with glucose, thus setting off the insulin-adrenalin regulatory mechanism, which may cause sudden rises and falls in the body's blood sugar, with resulting PMS symptoms such as anxiety, dizziness, headache and sugar craving.

Complex carbohydrates are not sweet to the taste, and are in the form of starches and dextrins. They cause a more controlled and slower rise of the blood sugar because of their slower breakdown time; thus the chances of an insulin-adrenalin reaction are greatly reduced.

Simple and Complex Carbohydrates

Some simple carbohydrates that increase PMS symptoms	Some complex carbohydrates that reduce PMS symptoms
White and refined bread Many highly refined convenience foods Carbonated sugared drinks	Whole grain, wholemeal and rye breads
Sweets Dried fruit	Cereals such as muesli and wholegrain types Wheat crackers
Very sweet fresh fruit Canned and frozen fruit Ice cream Sweet desserts and pies White and brown sugar Syrup, molasses and honey Young vegetables such as baby carrots and mange tout	Dried legumes (pulses) Pasta from wholemeal flour Potatoes Wheat crackers Brown and wild rice

Table 6

Generally speaking, the degree of ripeness of fruits and vegetables dictates the relative proportion of sugar and starch. Fresh, immature vegetables such as mange tout, baby carrots and sweet corn have less starch content and more sugar than mature vegetables and fruit: (Some varieties of apple – Newtons and Granny Smiths, for instance – contain less sugar than others; grapefruits contain less sugar than oranges.)

An exception to the rule is green and half-ripe bananas, which contain more starch and less sugar than ripe bananas, in which the sugar content is very high — and so should be avoided. Ripe bananas are also very rich in amines, which can cause severe headaches and depression in individuals who lack the necessary enzymes for breaking the amines down.

Low sugar recipes are included in Appendix C to help you control your simple carbohydrate intake.

4. Increase dietary fibre

Fibre is a complex carbohydrate which occurs in two types — the *digestible*, which is found in fruits and vegetables, and the *indigestible*, one source of which is the tough outer bran layers of whole grain cereals. Both types increase the bulk of the stool, thereby reducing constipation, often a troublesome complaint in PMS. Fibre also reduces water absorption from the bowel because of its 'holding ability'; this in turn reduces to some extent the oedema (increased tissue fluid) associated with PMS.

Digestible fibre activates the normal bacteria in the bowel; it swells and holds water, thus increasing the size or bulk of the stool. Indigestible fibre — such as bran — by its spongelike quality causes water to be held in the stool.

Main Sources of Fibre

Digestible fibre	Indigestible fibre
Cooked prunes Almonds, brazil nuts Beans Chick peas, mung beans, lentils, Red kidney beans Dried or mature peas Parsley leaves Cabbage, broccoli, spinach Potato skins Soya flour (low fat) Raw oatmeal	Oatmeal bread Raw wheat bran Raw oat bran Rye bread Bran cereal Wholegrain cereals

Table 7

Recently another fibre, *pectin*, an indigestible complex carbohydrate that swells with water and produces a gel, has been used to increase stool bulk and reduce constipation. Pectin is present in fruit, but because of the sweetness of many ripe fruits, they should be consumed only in small daily quantities. This also applies to dried fruit, where the sugar content can be even higher.

Caution in the use of bran fibre must be exercised because it can produce excess gas, cramping and malabsorption of some nutrients. A safe level of bran intake either as wheat bran or oat bran is approximately 20–30 g (2/3–1 oz.) daily, with *additional fibre* intake coming from fruits and vegetables.

5. Achieve adequate protein intake

Proteins are complex organic compounds constructed of amino acids. There are over 20 amino acids, and nine of them cannot be manufactured in the body. They are therefore termed *essential* and have to be ingested in the *food we eat*.

Some foods are *complete proteins*; examples are eggs, milk and meat, including fish and poultry. Other protein is *partially complete*; it will maintain life, but it lacks some amino acids necessary, for example, for growth. Such partially complete proteins occur in breads, cereals, beans, peas and peanut butter. When partial protein is supplemented with small amounts of complete protein, the complete protein intake — including expensive fresh meat — can be reduced, because the two combine and form a complete protein, which supplies the required amino acids for balanced protein nutrition.

Main Sources of Protein

Complete	Incomplete
Meat	Peanuts
Poultry	Bread
Fish	Beans
Cheese	Peas
Eggs	Potatoes
Milk	Rice
	Fruit
	Tofu

Table 8

Protein forms the solid matter of muscles, organs and endocrine glands. Enzymes are protein in nature, and so are

47

many hormones. PMS is in part a hormonal imbalance; therefore, it is very important to maintain an adequate dietary supply of the amino acids needed for protein formation. This can be achieved only with good and sensible nutrition.

Milk, while an excellent complete protein, can interfere with the absorption and utilization of essential fatty acids because of its own animal fat content. Milk also contains — along with cheese — a considerable amount of sodium; therefore, during the last two weeks of the menstrual cycle, reduce your intake of milk products. Soya milk is a healthy alternative.

6. Eat regularly and on time — never allow more than 3 hours to pass between meals.

7. Eat snacks of complex carbohydrates or protein between meals

By maintaining stable blood sugar levels, you can reduce PMS symptoms such as headache, irritability, nervousness and food craving that are attributed to fluctuating and low blood sugar levels. Do not go for long periods without eating. This produces a fall in your blood sugar levels and causes symptoms to occur. This rule applies not only during the pre-menstruum but all through the cycle. Try to have three balanced meals during the day, with emphasis on complex carbohydrates and protein, and a low intake of simple carbohydrates, especially sugars. Fats should comprise approximately 25 to 30 per cent of your calorie intake, with 80 per cent coming from vegetable oil (polyunsaturated) sources. Animal (saturated) fats should be kept to a minimum to reduce your cholesterol intake.

A small snack mid-morning, mid-afternoon and just before bed will also ensure blood sugar level stability. Such snacks may consist of, for example, a semi-ripe apple or perhaps a couple of thin wheat crackers or crispbreads, plain wheat biscuits and low-salt cheese. Usually peanut butter and wheat crackers with half a glass of skimmed milk before bed assists deep, satisfying sleep. Tofu may be substituted for peanut butter, since it too is rich in iron and calcium.

Because of the extreme sweetness of fructose (fruit sugar), it is wise to avoid very sweet fruit such as overripe fruit, tropical fruits like pineapple, and all dried fruit during the last two weeks of the menstrual cycle.

8. Add linoleic acid and gamma-linolenic acid to diet

The importance of linoleic acid (LA) in the production of prostaglandins is discussed in Chapter 3. In PMS a prostaglandin imbalance is thought to be present. To maintain adequate and balanced prostaglandins, the diet must be rich in essential fatty acids, the building blocks of prostaglandins, which are found in sunflower, safflower and corn oils. The most important essential fatty acid is LA in the *cis* form.

The conversion of LA to prostaglandins requires enzymes and certain nutrients (see Chart 5). The most important enzyme is delta-6-desaturase (D-6-D). Its efficiency can be thwarted or reduced by stress; diets rich in simple sugars or highly refined foods; a lack of nutrients such as vitamin B_6, vitamin C, magnesium and zinc; and diets high in processed vegetable oils as found in certain margarines, where the *trans* fatty acids block the D-6-D activity. As well, cancer, alcohol and diets rich in saturated (animal) fats reduce the formation of gamma-linolenic acid (GLA) from LA, a part of the conversion process, to the formation of prostaglandin E1.

Adequate intake of LA can prevent, or at least reduce, thwarting of the conversion process. It is possible to bypass the formation of GLA by ingesting it directly in the form of Efamol capsules, which contain the seed oil of the evening primrose (*oenethera biennis*). This oil contains 72 per cent cis-LA and approximately 10 per cent GLA. The dosage varies from woman to woman. The only side effect that I have found is occasional nausea, but this can be avoided by taking the capsules with food, and never on an empty stomach. If nausea persists, the capsule may be broken and the oil rubbed onto the skin of the abdomen or arms, where it will be rapidly absorbed. The oil has a softening effect on the stool, and the subsequent easing of constipation is welcomed by many with PMS for whom constipation is a frequent complaint.

1 capsule	daily with food from day 5 to day 10 of the cycle.
1 capsule twice	daily with food from day 11 to day 19 of the cycle.
1 capsule thrice	daily with food from day 20 to day 28 of the cycle.

This is an average dose schedule, but as with all preparations, even 'natural' ones such as this, fine alterations of dosage are required. Dosages are carefully assessed at follow-up visits or by telephone.

Finding your LA and GLA tolerance level

The level of nutrients that you require for the control of your PMS symptoms must be individualized to your needs. The dosage scheme outlined above is one I have found to be completely safe, and a helpful starting point. Caffeine restriction, sodium reduction, increase of fibre and alteration of carbohydrate and protein intake will all require little or no fine tuning, but are crucial to your overall improvement.

The GLA capsule dosage may have to be increased after the second month. If some improvement has occurred, then increase the dosage to three capsules each day, from day 11 to day 20 of the cycle. If, after another month, no further improvement has occurred, try increasing to four capsules each day (two in the morning and two in the evening) from day 20 to day 28 of the cycle, but leave the dosage at three capsules each day from day 11 to day 19 and two capsules daily from day 5 to day 10.

On the higher LA and GLA dosage regime, you may experience some slight nausea or looseness of bowel action. Take your capsules with food and do not worry. Reduce the dosage slightly until you find your own level of tolerance, or alter the time of day when you take the capsule. This fine tuning should overcome any problems. Very rarely have I had to increase a dosage to four capsules daily; usually, satisfactory response is obtained with the lower dosage levels.

I have found that if the key regime is carefully followed it is not always necessary to employ the LA/GLA capsule treatment. I always encourage my patients to *first try* taking the LA as vegetable oil, incorporating in the diet approximately two tablespoons of sunflower or safflower oil each day, in salads, cold dishes and by local application (rubbing into the skin). If sufficient D-6-D enzyme is available, formation of prostaglandins should take place.

The conversion process from LA to prostaglandins continues with GLA being processed to dihomogammalinolenic acid (DGLA). Other nutrients are necessary for this conversion (below).

9. Add necessary nutrients to diet

Crucial *assistance factors* for the prostaglandin manufacture from cis-LA are B-complex vitamins, vitamin B_6, vitamin C, calcium, magnesium and zinc.

B-complex vitamins

Just as D-6-D is the enzyme necessary to complete the conversion of LA to GLA, the B-complex vitamins, acting as co-enzymes, are required for many of the biochemical processes that eventually form prostaglandins. The water-soluble B-complex vitamins are grouped together and consist of eight structures. The first two of the group, thiamin and riboflavin, usually head any formula on a vitamin

B-complex list. Each of these should be in a dosage of 50 mg; the remaining six are in adequate relative proportions.

Example of B-complex Formula:

Thiamin	(B_1)	50 mg
Riboflavin	(B_2)	50 mg
Niacin	(B_3)	50 mg
Pyridoxine	(B_6)	50 mg
Pantothenic acid		50 mg
Biotin		100 mcg
Folic acid		5 mg
Vitamin B_{12}		50 mcg

Occasionally choline and inositol may be included, but their importance has not been established. Dosage is usually 1 tablet on alternate days.

Vitamin B_6 (pyridoxine)

In addition to the 50 mg in the B-complex formula, extra vitamin B_6 should be taken. Vitamin B_6 converts tryptophan to niacin. The activity of vitamin B_6 can be reduced by some drugs used in the treatment of tuberculosis, and more commonly by steroidal contraceptive pills. In such cases B_6 supplements are required.

Vitamin B_6 reduces the effect of prolactin. It is helpful in reducing many of the prolactin-associated symptoms of PMS, such as bloating, breast soreness and tenderness. Mood changes and headaches may also be greatly assisted.

The optimum dosage of B_6 has to be carefully evaluated on an individual basis. I usually start patients at 50 mg daily, in addition to the vitamin B_6 contained in the B-complex vitamin. This second dose is given at a different time to that of the B-complex and always with a meal, to avoid excess acidity. After one month the dosage may have to be increased by adding another 50 mg tablet either in the morning or evening. Fine tuning of the dosage takes place over the next two to three months. Once the correct dosage of vitamin B_6 has been found for you, it is continued for approximately nine months, and gradual reduction may then be attempted if symptoms have vanished. I usually advise that the dosage may be reduced by 25 mg each month. If symptoms reoccur, the dosage may be increased again. Toxicity to B_6 is rare, and symptoms usually occur with daily dosages above 150 mg. Symptoms may take the form of itching skin, extreme sensitivity of the breasts and vagina, and crawling sensations under the skin, particularly on the legs. Another caution: if a patient has Parkinson's disease and is being treated with Levodopa, vitamin B_6 will reverse the benefit of the medication.

Natural sources of vitamin B_6 are meat, poultry, fish, potatoes and vegetables.

Vitamin C (ascorbic acid)

Ascorbic acid is needed for prostaglandin formation. It also plays an important role in the strength of blood vessels, as well as in healing of the skin.

If you smoke or drink, your needs for vitamin C will be higher because these activities greatly reduce the body's ability to store ascorbic acid. Stress will also increase your vitamin C requirements.

In such cases I suggest 500 mg a day; otherwise 250 mg daily taken with food should be adequate. Usually the least expensive ascorbic acid tablets are as effective as the most expensive. Vitamin C is called the 'fresh food' vitamin, for it is in its highest natural concentration in fresh picked fruits and vegetables. Natural sources are citrus fruits, tomatoes, melons, cabbage, broccoli, strawberries, new potatoes and green leafy vegetables.

Folic acid

Women who take oral contraceptives show decreased folic acid blood levels. These levels do not appear to return to normal until about three months after the contraceptive medication has been stopped. A lowered folic acid blood level can give rise to megaloblastic anaemia; here the red blood cells become larger than they should be. It can also produce cell changes on the surface of the cervix (cervical dysplasia), the first evidence of which may be found in changes on a smear test. Emotional swings have been reported in women who have low folic acid blood levels during and after oral contraceptive use, thus aggravating PMS symptoms.

Calcium, magnesium and zinc

The mineral nutrients calcium, magnesium and zinc are vital for proper body function. They are essential for enzyme and co-enzyme action. They are required in the production of many hormones and for the transmission of electrical nerve impulses in muscles and organs. They also play an important role in blood clotting.

Calcium and magnesium compete with each other for absorption. Therefore, a higher intake of one may produce an imbalance. Both should be prescribed together, in the ratio of twice as much calcium as magnesium, since the body's requirement of calcium is far greater than that of magnesium.

Recent research has shown a link between magnesium lack and Toxic Shock Syndrome. Some tampons are thought to absorb excessive magnesium. Such a magnesium reduction may, in sensitive women, aggravate PMS symptoms.

Zinc is distributed widely but not uniformly in all body tissues. It is an important part of at least 20 enzymes; an example is carbonic anhydrase, which is essential for the transport of carbon dioxide to the lungs. Zinc aids in the building of DNA and RNA and therefore of protein. Very importantly, it is required for the satisfactory action of follicle stimulating and luteinizing hormones. A definite relationship has been shown between a mother's zinc level and the weight of her babies; it would appear that a mother's zinc level 20 per cent or more below normal can be associated with impaired foetal growth.

I have found the most beneficial daily dosage of the three mineral nutrients to be:

Calcium	500 mg
Magnesium	250 mg
Zinc	30 mg

Care should be taken in purchasing these mineral nutrients. Calcium from crushed oyster shell is excellent and comes in the form of calcium carbonate. Calcium is prevented from complete absorption by oxalic acid found in rhubarb and spinach and by phytic acid in bran and whole cereals. Do not take the calcium at the same time as these foods.

Natural Sources of Mineral Nutrients

Calcium	Magnesium	Zinc
Milk	Milk	Liver
Milk products	Cheese	Oysters
Green leafy vegetables	Green leafy vegetables	Beef
Canned salmon with bones	Dried beans and peas	Lamb
Shrimp	Soya beans	Pork
	Nuts	Dark meat of poultry
	Whole grains	Legumes
		Peanut butter

Table 9

Magnesium is usually taken as the oxide. Neither calcium nor magnesium should be taken within three hours of ingesting the antibiotic tetracycline, because either may reduce its absorption. I do not use dolomite as a source of magnesium because it may contain environmental contaminants such as heavy metals.

Zinc may be taken in either the sulphate or gluconate form. Its action is reduced by alcohol, diuretics and oral contraceptives. Zinc can interact negatively with other nutrients such as iron and copper, and should therefore be taken an hour or more away from meals.

10. Change lifestyle

Excess alcohol either during occasional 'binge drinking' or through daily intake can severely interfere with the absorption of essential nutrients such as vitamins and minerals. Alcohol-induced chronic liver disease, even in a low grade form, can alter the fat structure of the blood, producing an increase in triglycerides. This in turn can cause an inflammation of the pancreas and over time, affect the clotting mechanisms of the blood. Amino acids, zinc, potassium and magnesium are readily washed out of the body, in the urine. Such a loss puts at risk the fine biochemical mechanism that is required for prostaglandin and hormone manufacture. This will, of course worsen PMS symptoms. An occasional glass of dry red or white wine with a meal can be beneficial, but drinking should be kept at that level, and in the pre-menstruum you should abstain from alcohol entirely if you have PMS symptoms.

Stop smoking

Smoking is a proven risk to health. It causes arterial disease and lung cancer. It interferes with the transfer of oxygen to the blood in the lungs, worsening the tiredness, lethargy and irritability associated with PMS. There is a link between a mother's smoking and premature birth, due in part to poor placental development, with resulting lessening of nutrient and oxygen transfer to the developing foetus.

To stop smoking is a lifestyle change paramount in the overall treatment regime of PMS.

Stop oral contraceptives

Approximately 90 per cent of women who use or have used the birth control pill experience increased PMS symptoms. The symptoms most commonly reported are depression, headache and weight gain. Nausea and bloatedness are also frequently noticed symptoms.

It is thought that birth control pills reduce the body's ability to absorb vitamin B_6. Many of the symptoms can be reduced by taking extra vitamin B_6, as described earlier in this chapter.

This poor tolerance of the pill is probably due to the fact that the oestrogen-progestogen which it contains lowers the *plasma concentration of natural progesterone.*
Oestrogen-progestogen birth control pills now available are less likely to cause such severe problems because the potency of the hormone they contain is less. However, women who have troublesome PMS should come off the birth control pill entirely and use another form of contraception.

Manage stress through exercise and relaxation

Stress can be called the 'extension of strain'. Up to our maximal tolerance level, stress improves our performance and enjoyment of life by making us meet fair challenges. This is a healthy balance. (Too little challenge can produce imbalance in the form of 'burn-out'.) Each of us has different tolerance levels. Compare it to a thermostat: when the temperature and humidity level remain within defined upper and lower limits, we feel comfortable; outside these levels some distress occurs. Distress in life is caused by *stressors*, and these can be internal or external.

The key to reducing excess stress is to understand your own motives, ambitions, habits and weaknesses. By identifying your 'comfort zone', you will be able to recognize when you are moving out of it. By analyzing your lifestyle, you can make appropriate changes to reduce stress, and thereby lessen PMS symptoms, many of which are the direct cause of being outside your comfort zone.

In the overall treatment of PMS I evaluate stress in detail and use the following questionnaires to ascertain where the major stressors are. After this evaluation, a management and preventive approach to stress, which must be individualized to your needs, is begun. By completing these questionnaires, you will be able to judge if stress is affecting you to any significant level. After discussing the results with your doctor, he or she will know the problem. (The Life Events Questionnaire included in this book was developed by Thomas Holmes and Richard Rahe, psychiatrists at the University of Washington School of Medicine, U.S.A., in 1967.)

External and Internal Stressors

External stressors — environmental

— Type of job
— Unhappy marriage
— Other family problems
— Recent bereavement
— Too much to do and too little time in which to do things.
— Noise
— Crowding
— Rapid change
— Financial problems

Internal stressors — personal

— Perfectionism
— Oversensitivity
— Anger
— Guilt
— Fear
— Type 'A' personality (hard-driving, achievement-oriented, very competitive, time-urgent)

Life Events Questionnaire

	2 years	6 months
Death of a spouse	75	100
Divorce	63	84
Marital separation	51	70
Term of imprisonment	45	63
Death of a close family member	44	62
Personal injury or major illness	37	53
Marriage	34	50
Fired from work	32	47
Marital reconciliation	30	45
Retirement	30	45
Dental stress	75	75
Change in the health of a family member	29	45
Pregnancy	26	40
Sexual difficulties	25	39
Gain of a new family member	24	39

Business re-adjustment	24	39
Marriage of daughter	23	38
Change in financial state	22	38
Death of a close friend	21	37
Change to different line of work	21	36
Change in residence	20	36
Change in number of arguments with spouse	19	35
Very large mortgage	17	31
Foreclosure of mortgage or loan	16	30
Change in responsibilities at work	15	29
Marriage of son	15	29
Son or daughter leaving home	14	29
Trouble with in-laws	14	29
Outstanding personal achievement	13	28
Spouse begins or stops work	12	26
Begin or end school	11	25
Change in schools	11	25
Revision of personal habits	10	24
Trouble with boss	8	21
Change in sleeping habits	8	21
Change in work hours or conditions	8	20
Change in recreation	7	19
Change in church activities	7	19
Change in social activities	6	18
Small mortgage or large personal loan	6	17
Change in number of family get-togethers	5	15
Change in eating habits	5	15
Vacation	4	13
Large celebration (e.g. Christmas)	4	12
Minor violations of the law	3	11

Instructions: Circle the point of values that apply to you. Be careful to use the correct column according to when the event took place. Add up your score. If your total exceeds 300, then you are overstressed and have a 50 per cent chance of experiencing a stress-related illness. Between 200 and 300 indicates moderate stress, and you have approximately a 30 per cent chance of experiencing some physical symptoms. A score of under 200 indicates that minor stress is present, but you should be able to handle it without problems.

Is Stress Affecting You?

In the last *two months* I have had or experienced:

	1 2 3 4
Tension headache	1 2 3 4
Fatigue	1 2 3 4
Constipation	1 2 3 4
Muscle cramps or spasms; jaw tension	1 2 3 4
Low back pain or any chronic pain	1 2 3 4
High blood pressure	1 2 3 4
Hives	1 2 3 4
Low grade infections	1 2 3 4
Indigestion	1 2 3 4
Hyperventilation (breathing irregularities)	1 2 3 4
Dermatitis	1 2 3 4
Menstrual problems	1 2 3 4
Nausea or vomiting	1 2 3 4
Migraine headaches	1 2 3 4
Loss of appetite	1 2 3 4
Diarrhoea	1 2 3 4
Aching neck and shoulder muscles	1 2 3 4
Asthma attack	1 2 3 4
Colitis attack	1 2 3 4
Arthritis	1 2 3 4
Common flu or cold	1 2 3 4
Metabolic disorder: diabetes; thyroid	1 2 3 4
Peptic ulcer	1 2 3 4
Cold hands or feet or excess perspiration	1 2 3 4
Heart palpitations	1 2 3 4
Dizziness	1 2 3 4

Instructions: Use the following scale: 1 = Never, 2 = Occasionally, 3 = Frequently, 4 = Constantly. Add up your score. A score between 35 and 50 is average. If the score is nearer to 50, then it is very probable that a life event or personal change may have occurred that could have affected your general health.

Stress Self-Assessment

Instructions: tick the appropriate column in the following table if you have been bothered by that stress-related problem.

During the past *one month* I have:	Never	Once in a while	Fairly often	Very often
Had trouble remembering things				
Had my mind go blank				
Become angry over unimportant things				
Felt critical of others				
Had irrational fear or outright panic				
Felt lonely				
Felt easily annoyed or irritated				
Had difficulty making decisions				
Lost interest in sex				
Lost my temper				
Thought about ending my life				
Felt scared or afraid				
Had trouble concentrating				
Had to avoid something or someone because I was scared				
Felt hopeless about the future				
Felt tense, agitated or 'keyed up'				
Felt loss of self-confidence				
Been eating too much or lost my appetite				
Been sleeping too much or too little				
Cried easily or felt like crying				
Consumed more alcohol or non-prescription drugs than I'd like				
Been in minor accidents (car or other)				
Used prescription drugs				
Driven recklessly				
Developed or been subject to mannerisms — nail biting, toe tapping, hair twisting, muscle twitches				
Had insatiable cravings (food, etc.)				
Been clumsy or shaky				

To achieve stress control and reduce the undesirable effects of stress, it is important to:

- Have a balanced lifestyle, providing acceptable time for yourself, work, family life, hobbies, sport and exercise. Ask yourself what you can stop doing.
- Know yourself well, including your ambitions, desires and the limits of your comfort zone.
- Maintain good physical health, with a well-balanced diet, adequate sleep, and regular exercise.
- Set yourself achievable and worthwhile short- and long-term goals. This will give you a sense of purpose and direction.
- Have a belief system. Remember that if you say 'I think I can,' often enough it becomes 'I know I can,' and then 'I knew I could.'
- Have friendship and fellowship. Above all, your partner in life should be a 'good friend'.
- Maintain and improve your sense of humour.
- Attend an assertiveness training group to assist you to cope with the excessive demands of others.

It is not the intention of this book to describe *in detail* stress management techniques. However, I will briefly discuss various methods that have been very helpful, in my own practice, for the reduction of stress. (See the Bibliography for further reading.)

The hallmark of many stress management techniques is *relaxation*. This form of therapy can be achieved by four methods:

1. Focussing your attention on an object or other focal point, and breathing in and out slowly and evenly.
2. Using muscle group relaxation, by progressively tensing, then relaxing, groups of muscles in a patterned way.
3. Mental imagery, by concentrating on a soothing or relaxing scene.
4. Standard Autogenic Training (SAT).

The first three methods are self-explanatory, but SAT deserves explanation. Standard Autogenic Training was originally developed by J.W. Schultz in Germany and is widely used in Europe as well as in Japan and North America, where it has come to the forefront of stress management during the last ten years. The method involves training an individual in six standard exercises. Involved is the feeling of warmth and heaviness in the extremities of the body, a feeling of coolness about the forehead, with warmth perceived in the abdomen. This, along with slow, deep breathing and reduced heart action, creates long-term conditioning of the nervous system. The 'flight and fight' response to stress is replaced by the calmer, controlled relaxation response.

SAT has been shown to significantly improve feelings of tension and depression. I have found it to be very helpful in the overall treatment of PMS, proving that stress can be altered by behavioural modification.

Exercise is also beneficial in the control and alteration of stress. It improves the cardiovascular system, strengthens the heart muscle and reduces the harmful effects of low density cholesterol by inversely increasing the level of the protective high density cholesterol in the blood. Exercise also improves oxygen supply to the brain, its muscle action massages certain organs, and it causes better nutrient absorption from the intestine, because of improved and more rapid blood supply. A word of caution: before you embark on an exercise programme, get a medical evaluation and physical examination done, to establish the health and strength of your cardiovascular system, your spine, and your ankle and knee joints.

Society today is obsessed with thinness. Eating disorders such as anorexia nervosa and bulimia are often linked with menstrual disorders. Severe weight loss caused by both these medical problems results in reduced hypothalamic influence, causing a reduction in the luteinizing and follicle stimulating hormones from the pituitary gland. Menstrual periods may stop completely, and the lack of oestrogen can cause a serious loss of bone calcium, resulting in early osteoporosis.

Excessive exercise causes similar hormonal level changes, absence of menstruation and alteration of hormonal balance. Moderation is very important in exercise. Enough is good, too much is harmful; therefore, a sensible approach should be employed. It is also important that any exercise programme should be fun, and that you should look forward to exercising. Set a certain time aside each day — the mornings are usually the best, when you are at your freshest, but that will depend upon your lifestyle and working schedule.

Always begin a programme slowly, perhaps 5 to 10 minutes to start, and gradually work up to one hour each day. Try to vary the type of exercise that you do. Use your own music recordings or participate in your favourite TV fitness programme. By exercising to the music you find agreeable, you will enjoy the exercise and you will put more enthusiasm into it.

Calisthenics can be done at any time of the day when you may need a boost, and include sit-ups, knee bends, toe touching, arm circles, head rotating, side bends, arm twists, knee-ups and leg lifts. Appendix E outlines a group of excellent exercises especially contrived by a prima ballerina to help stress reduction and weight loss.

The object of *aerobics* is to raise the heart rate to around 120 beats per minute for a short period — 15 to 20 minutes — about three or four times weekly. Start out for 3 to 4 minutes only and take perhaps 10 to 15 weeks to reach your goal. Aerobic activities such as jumping, dancing, kicking and skipping exercise specific muscle groups and improve general flexibility.

Aerobic classes have become very popular. A typical class lasts for 45 to 60 minutes approximately, three times weekly. Ideally the time should consist of a 10 to 15 minute warm-up of stretching exercise similar to calisthenics, followed by 15 to 20 minutes of sustained high-intensity aerobic activity, often called cardiovascular exercise because the heart and its action is the principal target of the exercise pattern. This should be followed by 10 to 15 minutes of cool-down exercises. The class is directed by an instructor who leads the group in time to recorded dance music.

To reduce possible aerobic class injury you should:
- Select an instructor and organization with a good programme and reputation.
- Start slowly and gradually increase your exercise time.
- Choose a good pair of cushioned, supportive exercise shoes.
- Have adequate warm-up and cool-down periods.
- Have periodic safety monitoring and pulse checks during the workout.

Other excellent forms of aerobic exercise are fast walking, swimming, bicycling and racquet sports. Fast walking is probably the best and safest exercise of all. It imposes only about a third of the impact stress on the knees compared to jogging. However, the most likely cause of injury is pushing yourself beyond a pleasant level of tiredness. The possibility of injury is increased tenfold by the element of severe competition. Remember to start slowly and pace yourself.

There are now many *relaxation* techniques, often based on techniques which originated in the East, that are beneficial in reducing stress. I only list them here; specific texts should be consulted for further detailed reading.

Oriental medicine believes in life energy called *Chi*, which is distributed throughout the body by way of meridian channels. The areas where these channels surface are the acupressure points. Acupuncture refers to the insertion of needles into these points to increase the flow of energy.

Acupressure is the use of thumb or finger pressure to create the same effect as the needle. *Shiatsu* is a similar form of therapy to acupressure and originated in Japan.

Yoga is an excellent form of relaxation that emphasizes the importance of posture, breathing and meditation. The exercises are most helpful. In the hands of an expert teacher, yoga can greatly relieve PMS.

The *Alexander Technique* is a form of therapy that requires you to attend instructional classes. Its premise is that symptoms of stress and strain can be controlled and improved by correcting body alignment and poor posture.

The Chinese art of *Tai Chi* requires you to attend classes for instruction. Grace and poise are married to rhythmical movement of muscle and limb, producing relaxation of tension and a quietening of the mind. Tai Chi teaches relaxation in the face of conflict, rather than reaction to conflict in the form of stress or illness.

Reflexology is a technique of foot massage that originated in China over two thousand years ago. Like acupressure and shiatsu, it shares the same philosophy of energy fields and stress points. In reflexology, manipulation and pressure of the feet relieve tension and stress.

Perhaps the most universal method of relaxation is *body massage*. Certainly in the skilled hands of a professional therapist, massage can be greatly relaxing.

Part II: Severe PMS

Probably no more than 5 per cent of women require treatment for PMS by other than the ten-point key regime. These 5 per cent of women with severe PMS usually fit into one or more of the following categories:

- Those whose symptoms have not been relieved by diet or lifestyle changes.
- Those with upsetting recurrent symptoms that may interfere with their ability to work or upset marital harmony.
- Those with pre-menstrual symptoms that cause recurrent bouts of alcohol abuse, assault, injury or criminal offences.

Sufferers from severe PMS are so affected by the severity of their symptoms that they are unable to function normally. Depression, panic or violence may be so overwhelming that family life is drastically altered. Criminal offences may be committed, and bodily injury may result.

Treatment of those suffering from severe PMS requires the key regime to be started as detailed in Part I of this chapter and continued as summarized in Chart 10 (page 64). The key regime is supplemented by one or more of the following treatment options. The use of progesterone is an option that is both helpful and effective.

Summary of Key Regime

NO CAFFEINE
REDUCE SALT (SODIUM) IN THE DIET ↓
REDUCE SIMPLE CARBOHYDRATE INTAKE ↓
INCREASE COMPLEX CARBOHYDRATE AND
DIETARY FIBRE ↑
EAT MEALS REGULARLY AND ON TIME
SNACK BETWEEN MEALS WITH COMPLEX
CARBOHYDRATE OR PROTEIN
ADEQUATE PROTEIN CONSUMPTION

ESSENTIAL FATTY ACIDS
LINOLEIC ACID OR GAMMA-
LINOLENIC ACID IN THE FORM OF
CORN OIL, SUNFLOWER,
SAFFLOWER OR
EFAMOL CAPSULES (GLA CAPSULES)

INCREASE ↑

DECREASE ↓

NECESSARY NUTRIENTS
VITAMIN C
VITAMIN B_6
VITAMIN B-COMPLEX
CALCIUM
MAGNESIUM
ZINC

LIFESTYLE CHANGE
REDUCE ALCOHOL CONSUMPTION
STOP SMOKING
STOP ORAL CONTRACEPTIVES
STRESS MANAGEMENT
RELAXATION
EXERCISE

Chart 10

I have found it possible to achieve an 80 per cent satisfactory improvement rate in controlling the severe symptoms of PMS by using one or a combination of the options below. In treating *all* cases of severe PMS, however, I remove from the diet *amine-rich* foods. A build-up of amines in the body interferes with the action of neurotransmitters such as dopamine, noradrenaline and serotonin. A malfunctioning of neurotransmitters is responsible for the worsening of depression and increasing of prolactin blood levels. Depression and prolactin are closely involved in the symptoms of PMS.

Table 11: Severe PMS Treatment Summary

1. The key regime.
2. Remove amine-rich foods from diet, as listed in Table 2. Additional options include treatment by:
3. Diuretics
4. Anti-depressants
5. Bromocriptine
6. Danazol
7. Progesterone — natural and synthetic.

Diuretics
If the severe symptoms that have not been relieved by diet or lifestyle changes are those of fluid retention, then a potassium-sparing diuretic such as Spironolactone (Aldactone) may be given in dosages of 50 mg and 25 mg on alternate days, from ovulation to the onset of menstruation. I have found satisfactory results with this method in some women with persistent and severe water retention.

It is always wise to have the serum potassium level checked if the use of this selective diuretic has to be continued for more than three months.

Anti-depressants
Depression is a common symptom in severe PMS, but treatment with anti-depressant drugs has not been very successful. In women suffering from PMS, depression may be linked to prolactin production by the pituitary gland. Unfortunately one of the most useful anti-depressant groups, the tricyclic group, of which Aventyl, Elavil and Tofranil are members, causes an increase of prolactin and a lowering of progesterone blood levels, causing worsening of other PMS symptoms such as bloating and lethargy. After taking the drugs there can be a delay of seven to ten days until benefit occurs; it is necessary to take them when menstruation begins

in order to achieve the benefit when it is needed — after ovulation has taken place and this is not very practical.

Another group of anti-depressants, often referred to as mono-amine oxidase inhibitors (MAOs), is more beneficial. These drugs (for example Parnate and Nardil), because their use requires severe restriction of certain foods to avoid side effects, are also impractical for treatment of PMS generally. But because of their short delay action (one to two days) they have been used for severe cyclical depression in the pre-menstruum: MAOs are administered each month for a few days when depression is most troublesome, and are discontinued when menstruation begins.

Bromocriptine

The neurotransmitter dopamine exerts a braking effect on the hypothalamus. When this happens, the hypothalamus activates the pituitary gland to produce prolactin in greater or lesser amounts, according to the level of dopamine present. Bromocriptine works against dopamine, reducing the amount of prolactin in the blood and therefore reducing prolactin-related PMS symptoms such as bloating, breast discomfort and lethargy. Unfortunately fluid retention, mood swings and irritability are not greatly relieved.

Bromocriptine is an extremely powerful drug; the usual starting dose is 2.5 mg daily (1.25 mg with breakfast and with supper). Nausea and vomiting are the main side effects, as well as dizziness due to the fall in blood pressure. The dosage has to be very carefully tuned to the patient's need and tolerance.

Bromocriptine is a derivative of ergot, a fungus, so it should not be used if any sensitivity to ergot exists. Alcohol should be avoided while this drug is being taken, and also great care should be employed if a patient is on blood pressure reducing medication.

Recently bromocriptine has been effective in reducing the acute symptoms of cocaine withdrawal. It was found that prolactin levels in chronic cocaine users were much higher, and dopamine levels lower. Bromocriptine in this case seems to counter the dopamine loss.

Danazol

This very powerful synthetic hormone has the ability to cause the pituitary gland to greatly reduce its release of FSH and LH, thereby putting the ovary to sleep, with a consequent halt of the menstrual cycle. Mood swings, so characteristic of the menstrual cycle, are eliminated. Danazol has limited value in the treatment of PMS, though in some areas it can be beneficial: it can relieve very severe cases of breast discomfort and extreme mood changes; endometriosis can be improved, and in some women completely suppressed; so too can the severe pain associated with extensive fibrocystic breast disease.

The dosage varies from 300 mg to 500 mg daily. Side effects include fluid retention, acne and nausea.

Progesterone — synthetic and natural

The hormone progesterone is necessary for the manufacture of various other hormones such as oestrogens, testosterone and the adrenal steroids. The peak level of progesterone normally occurs between day 20 and day 24 in the menstrual cycle. The symptoms of PMS coincide with this time in the cycle and reflect the difference in balance between oestrogen and progesterone. Synthetic progesterone (called progestogen), acts in the body like progesterone, with a few differences. Progesterone, for instance, causes a lessening of sodium and water retention, while progestogens cause the reverse.

Progestogens stop ovulation, and this is why these substances are an ingredient of the birth control pill. One of the synthetic progestogens, named dydrogesterone, is so close to the chemical structure of progesterone that it does not stop ovulation, nor does it have some of the masculinizing effects of the other progestogens. In the treatment of severe PMS where the addition of drug therapy is necessary my personal choice is natural progesterone. I have found it most beneficial in women with severe water retention or behaviour problems, and also in those with symptoms of depression and irritability, although there is little improvement in headaches. Two side effects can be nausea and increased breast discomfort.

Your doctor may be willing to try this medication for you, since it is considerably less expensive than natural progesterone, and has the benefit of being taken by mouth. The usual dose is 10 mg twice daily with meals, from day 12 to day 26 of the 28-day cycle. For women with shorter or longer cycles, the drug will have to be started earlier or later to give maximum benefit. Further fine-tuning of dosage may be required after a month.

A distinct disadvantage of *natural progesterone* is that it cannot be taken by mouth. It is also expensive. However, in cases where all other methods have been unsuccessful in treating severe PMS, natural progesterone should certainly be tried. It is important to continue the dietary alterations and lifestyle changes at the same time, as detailed in the key regime.

Before starting on progesterone, it is important that you know your menstrual cycle history. Your doctor will no doubt wish to see a chart of your cycle, with your symptoms clearly marked, to identify and reaffirm the diagnosis.

Natural progesterone may be given by rectal suppository, vaginal suppository, intramuscular injection or local implantation. In Britain administration in spray or gel form by the nasal route (where the drug is absorbed through the mucous membranes of the nose), is now being perfected. There are no serious side effects to natural progesterone; it is not carcinogenic, there are no addiction risks, there are no contra-indications to its use and there are no known drug interactions. Indeed, some drugs already being taken, such as anti-depressants and asthma-assisting medications, may even be reduced. (The vehicle or base with which the progesterone is combined in a suppository may cause irritation or burning. This can usually be overcome by changing to a suppository with a cocoa butter base.)

Sometimes troublesome yeast infection (*candidiasis*) may flare up when the drug is administered by the vaginal or rectal route, causing itching and irritation. The problem can be overcome by inserting and applying locally an anti-fungal preparation such as Nystatin or Clotrimazole before inserting the suppository. Possible leakage can be prevented by using a protective pad or by administering the suppository in divided dosages — two or three times daily instead of once daily.

In women who have not borne children, the starting dosage is one 400 mg suppository daily. In women who have borne children, the starting dosage is a 400 mg suppository twice daily. These are given either vaginally or rectally. Higher doses of progesterone are needed by women who have borne more than three children, who have suffered from depression following childbirth or who are underweight or slender in build.

The starting and stopping times of progesterone treatment depend upon your cycle length. When using progesterone suppositories, the administration usually begins at ovulation, with the beginning of your symptoms; the ending of the dosage is at menstruation. For example, if the menstrual cycle is short (22 days), progesterone should be started on day 9 of the cycle, or when ovulation occurs, and should be continued until menstruation begins.

If the menstrual cycle is long (36 days), start progesterone on day 21 and continue for only seven days. Menstruation may occur within 48 hours, thus reducing the cycle length to 30 days and avoiding the development of worsening symptoms.

If pre-menstrual symptoms last only for four days, but are very severe, in a 28-day cycle progesterone should be started on day 22 (two days before suspected onset of symptoms) and should be continued until menstruation begins.

Because progesterone is rapidly absorbed, reaching its blood level peak in about four hours and then falling over the next eight hours, the dosage may have to be split for better individual symptom control. For example, it may be better to adiminister one half of a 400 mg rectal suppository twice daily rather than one 400 mg suppository once daily. Such dosage alterations would be worked out by your doctor, dependent upon what is happening to your symptoms.

Fine tuning of the progesterone dosage is always required; it is therefore essential that you keep in close touch with your doctor. With so many variations in length of the menstrual cycle, and in the range of progesterone levels needed to control symptoms, sometimes daily phone calls between you and your doctor are necessary. If after using the suppositories for the second month you are symptom free, the daily dosage may be reduced from 400 mg to 200 mg. The time of starting the suppositories may also be delayed, so that in a 28-day cycle you now start on day 16 instead of day 14, depending upon when in the cycle your symptoms become troublesome. If only partial improvement has taken place, the dosage may be increased from one suppository to two, taken morning and evening. If you find your symptoms are worse in the evening than in the morning, the suppositories may be divided, allowing you to take one and a half in the evening and the other half in the morning.

Progesterone by injection is only required when suppositories prove unsuccessful due to patient dislike or from poor absorption of the drug. Progesterone by injection may well be the method of choice when a patient has to be hospitalized because of, for example, alcoholism or potential suicide.

Administration by implant may be a personal choice for those who have had good results taking progesterone in other ways. Implants are compressed pellets of natural progesterone which are placed in the fatty tissue of the tummy wall at yearly intervals, thus eliminating the need for injections or suppositories. Implants produce a continuous supply of progesterone. In some women this may alter the normal menstrual flow, but there is the advantage of prolonged control of PMS symptoms. Implants are sometimes used by those who have had a hysterectomy yet still find cyclical PMS troublesome or in alcoholics and those with poor memory.

Chapter 6

Additional Factors Affecting PMS

There are three conditions that may be confused with PMS because some of their symptoms are similar to those of PMS. The conditions are Candida albicans infection, food allergy symptoms and food additive reactions. These conditions may occur singly or in combination with each other.

Whereas PMS symptoms occur cyclically, beginning during the latter phase of the menstrual cycle and ending abruptly with onset of menstruation, symptoms from any of the above conditions can occur throughout the whole of the cycle and often worsen during the pre-menstruum. Oral antibiotics can destroy some of the naturally occurring bacteria in the bowel. When this happens, the naturally occurring yeasts that are also present tend to multiply. Vitamin synthesis is reduced and the hormone balance is disturbed, contributing further to symptoms of PMS.

Candida Albicans

Yeast infection is ubiquitous, occurring naturally on most body surfaces such as skin, lining of the intestine, mouth, vagina and rectum. This makes quantitative testing for yeast difficult and unreliable. Under certain circumstances, this 'living together' relationship between the yeast and its host becomes unbalanced, with increased yeast growth and resulting symptoms.

The toxins produced by the yeast organism are responsible for many of the typical symptoms. It is probable that yeast overgrowth severely worsens PMS. Yeast toxins can also alter the immune system. Allergy symptoms worsen when yeast symptoms increase; conversely, a decrease in symptoms occurs when yeast problems are controlled.

If you feel that you have a yeast problem, see your doctor. The treatment programme can be quite lengthy — usually three months — but your feeling of improvement makes the treatment worthwhile.

The treatment programme is individualized for each patient. I have had success using the virtually non-toxic drug Nystatin — which kills yeast on contact in the digestive tract — along with a rigid dietary change to cut off the nourishment yeast cells require.

Nystatin is available as a white powder in capsule form. It is taken by mouth, with water, on an empty stomach, one hour before a meal.

The starting dose has to be carefully individualized, and may be as small as one quarter of a capsule for the first two or three days, with increasing doses thereafter up to a maximum of three whole capsules each day.
Suggested Nystatin dosage follows:
1/4 capsule of powder daily for 3 days.
1/4 capsule of powder 3 times daily for 7 days.
1/2 capsule of powder 3 times daily for 7 days.
3/4 capsule of powder 3 times daily for 7 days.
1 capsule of powder 3 times daily for 6 weeks.

For the first ten days of treatment, mix the Nystatin powder with water and swish it around your mouth for a minute or two before swallowing. This will destroy any Candida in your mouth and throat.

Causes and Symptoms of Yeast Overgrowth

Causes
_____ Frequent or prolonged antibiotic use
_____ Cortisone-type medications
_____ Birth control pills
_____ Typical diet (too much sugar and refined foods)
Symptoms
_____ Vaginal discharge or itching
_____ Repeated attacks of cystitis (bladder infections)
_____ Constipation or diarrhoea, often alternating
_____ Excess gas and abdominal bloating
_____ Changes in menstrual cycle and flow
_____ Reduced libido and tiredness
_____ Altered emotions
_____ Depression, anxiety, irritability
_____ Loss of self-confidence

Table 12

During the first ten days of Nystatin treatment, improved destruction of the yeast takes place when the bowel acidity is increased. This is made possible by taking, by mouth, Lactobacillus acidophilus capsules — one capsule twice daily with food.

To maintain potency, the capsules should be stored in a

refrigerator at 10° C or below. Often a slight worsening of symptoms occurs during the initial phase of treatment. This is not a drug reaction but is a result of extra toxins having been released from the killed yeast cells. Such a worsening confirms the diagnosis.

Often yeast infection is present in the vagina as well as in the bowel. This can be diagnosed by your doctor by taking a vaginal swab. Vaginal yeast infections can be easily treated by using Nystatin vaginal suppositories or cream, or a similar antifungal product such as Clotrimazole or Miconazole.

Food to Avoid and Use in Treating Yeast Infections

Foods to Avoid

1. *All sweet foods:*
   Sugars
   Honey
   Molasses
   Maple syrup
   Corn syrup
   Carob

2. *All yeast-containing foods:*
   Baked goods with yeast
   Wines
   Beer, cider
   Other fermented beverages
   Yeast supplements and
   vitamins with a yeast base
   Breads raised with yeast

3. *Fermented extracts:*
   All cheese

   All vinegars
   Non-herbal teas

4. *All Fruit, nuts and mushrooms*

Foods You May Use

Very small amounts of:
Aspartame (artificial sweetener)

Unleavened breads and rye crispbreads
Baking powder sparingly in place of yeast

Cottage cheese or ricotta (made by curdling and not by fermentation)
Lemon juice in place of vinegar
Herbal teas
Low carbohydrate vegetables such as lettuce, spinach, broccoli, marrow, cauliflower, cucumbers and asparagus

Table 13

72

Nystatin will kill approximately 80 per cent of the Candida overgrowth; to complete treatment, it is necessary to stop eating the foods that nourish yeast cells. Basically, moulds and simple carbohydrates are eliminated from the diet. (These dietary changes are only temporary; a slow reintroduction of a regular diet can usually take place after about three months.)

The skin is also a site upon which yeast overgrowth can occur, and this should not be overlooked during the treatment. As yeast overgrowth prefers an alkaline medium (most soaps), the skin should be cleaned with acid-based soaps such as Neutragena. Local application of topical antifungal creams, especially to troublesome areas such as armpits, below the breasts, the groin, between the toes and on the feet, can produce excellent results. Examples of such creams are Nystatin, Canesten and Monistat.

With appropriate medication and diet, the improvement that can be achieved in the symptoms of PMS if you are also affected by Candida overgrowth can be very encouraging. It is an aspect of your overall treatment picture which should not be overlooked.

Allergy

Women with PMS are often atopic; in other words, they have a family tendency to allergic reactions such as rhinitis, eczema and asthma. Reactions that result may produce any or all of the following: breathlessness and throat constriction; marked fall in blood pressure; abdominal cramps, vomiting or diarrhoea; skin rashes (hives, nettle rash); asthma and eczema.

Prostaglandin production is crucial to the adequate protective functioning of the immune system. If prostaglandins are not in balance, this system breaks down, and an individual is more liable to react in an allergic way to triggering factors such as environmental pollutants and certain foods. This explains why a woman who has PMS symptoms is often found to have allergy symptoms as well.

If you suffer from asthma, hives or abdominal upsets that occur soon after eating, try to pinpoint which food is causing the reaction. Usually food allergy follows very quickly after the offending item is eaten. It is common for one group of symptoms, such as nausea and vomiting, to be accompanied by another, such as headache, weakness or skin rash. Such an occurrence should be reported to your doctor at once. If you believe that allergies are compounding your PMS symptoms with headaches, asthma or irritability, discuss this with your doctor so that appropriate testing can be done.

Tests will reveal what you are allergic to; thereby the offending 'allergen' in a particular food, hair spray, vapour and so on can be tracked down. It is often seen that a cross-sensitivity exists between common foods and inhalants: for example, a person with a detected tobacco or pollen allergy has an increased likelihood of reaction to milk, coffee, cocoa, chocolate or corn. In other words, the tobacco-sensitive individual may have an irritable bowel, or be prone to migraine attacks secondary to hidden reactions which are triggered by the ingestion of these foods. Similarly, patients with a grass pollen allergy may react to food 'grasses' such as wheat, cane sugar and rice.

Foods listed in Appendix A are grouped in families. If you are found to be allergic to a certain food family, then the associated members of the family should also be excluded from the diet, because 'triggering' of symptoms caused by another member of the family may occur.

If you suffer from coeliac disease you will, of course, know that gluten, an ingredient of wheat, must be excluded from your diet. Many pharmaceutical products contain gluten which is used as a binding agent, so if you do have coeliac disease you are advised to consult your doctor concerning the composition of any medication you are taking. The bloating associated with PMS may be worsened if gluten is present in any medication you take. Coeliac disease can also produce a marked reduction in the absorption of essential nutrients from the bowel, especially folate, iron, magnesium, calcium and zinc. Such a nutrient lack can aggravate the symptoms of PMS.

If you suspect you are sensitive to one of the main food groupings of milk, wheat or corn, rotational elimination is recommended. Take out of your diet for a period of seven to ten days all the milk-related products. If there is no improvement in your symptoms, remove all wheat and wheat products from your diet for the next seven to ten days, and return to taking milk and milk products. Then treat corn and corn products in the same way. By consulting Appendix A, you will discover which food group is causing your reaction.

Food allergies may produce a medical emergency requiring immediate skilled help. A Medic-Alert bracelet or neck chain identifying your sensitivity should be worn at all times. Your doctor will advise you where these can be obtained.

Food intolerance is another type of reaction. Here the body response is usually singular — a single reaction to a single food. Examples are: rapid heart action from caffeine; headaches due to wine, over-ripe cheese or cocoa; splitting of the red blood cells (haemolytic anaemia) due to eating fava beans.

Foods may also have a behavioural or emotional effect. For example, caffeine stimulates; alcohol depresses; sugars and refined carbohydrates can cause anxiety and irritability; food colouring has been implicated in hyperactivity in children.

Food Additives

Our bodies have not been able to adapt to all the nutritional changes that our packaged, preserved and 'chemicalized' environment has demanded of them. Our immune system is being overloaded with demands and attacks. We ourselves are causing many of the allergic reactions and emotional effects our bodies experience with all the foreign substances we present to our systems and expect them to cope with. To our insistence that food be appealing to the eye and have long keeping ability yet still retain its flavour and texture, high technology has responded with food additives. For the safety of each one of us, it is crucial that we understand food additives and know what is required for our protection.

Additives used to be listed under their category names only — artificial colour, for instance. The European Economic Community has now standardized food additives. Each has been given an 'E' number and a numerical code. The ingredient list on packaged foods must include these additive codes or the additive's specific chemical name. A consumer is therefore able to consult a handy reference guide that identifies the 'E' number and explains what the additive is, what it does and what side effects it may have.

Red dye No. 2 (Amaranth) was banned in the United States in 1976 but is still allowed in Canada and some other countries. Red dye No. 3 (Erythrocine), a synthetic coal tar derivative used in canned fruit and fruit pie filling, has been rated 1B by the World Health Organization, meaning that not enough data is available to make it completely acceptable for use in food. Red dye No. 3 has adverse effects on blood, and gene mutation has also been suspected. Because it contains 577 mg of iodine per gram, excess consumption of it could lead to hyperthyroidism (overactive thyroid). Red dye No. 3 can also produce increased sensitivity to light, with resulting skin rashes, and perhaps nausea.

It is vital and necessary for our protection that more detailed information be given on product labels about the additives they contain. Additives can cause many symptoms in people sensitive to them. A few of the many reactions are:

asthma, headache, nausea and vomiting, abdominal distension, skin rashes, swelling, numbness of mouth, irritability, mood swings, blurred vision, insomnia, vitamin deficiency, and digestive disturbances due to enzyme blockade. As well, additives may possibly be carcinogenic. Evidently, some of the reactions aggravate existing PMS symptoms. Therefore, it is important to be aware of what you are eating and try to consume as few additives as possible.

Not all food additives are necessarily dangerous, however. Some additives halt or prevent the growth in food of micro-organisms and bacteria. When food must spend time travelling from producer to consumer, for consumer protection some additives are necessary to keep the food safe for consumption. For example, sodium nitrite prevents the growth of Clostridium botulinum, the organism responsible for botulism. The addition of sodium ascorbate to bacon blocks the formation of nitrosamines a breakdown product of nitrites — which have been shown to be carcinogenic in animals but, as yet, not in man. This example demonstrates the fine balance that exists between the hazards of food additives and the hazards of unprotected foods; the risk factors present on both sides have to be weighed very carefully. Japan and Germany have banned nitrates and nitrites as food preservatives, judging them harmful and cancer-associated.

Potentially Harmful Colouring Agents

Substance	Action	Possible Side Effects
Tartrazine	Yellow colouring	Bronchospasm, skin rashes, blurred vision, insomnia
Sunset Yellow	Yellow colouring	Skin rash, vomiting, oedema, irritability
Caramel	Brown colouring	Vitamin B_6 deficiency suspected
Indigo carmine	Blue colouring	Nausea, hypertension, skin rash, itching, irritability

Table 14

The main food additive groups are:
– Colouring agents
– Preservatives
– Antioxidants
– Solvents
– Emulsifiers and stabilizers

Colouring agents make a product more eye-appealing. Some are natural, such as chlorophyll and saffron; many are synthetic, called *azo-dyes*, and may be hazardous. Azo-dyes cause sensitivity in about 20 per cent of people who are sensitive to aspirin. Azo-dye sensitivity may cause asthma, eczema, blurred vision, blood problems and, in extreme cases, shock.

Potentially Harmful Preservatives

Substance	Action	Possible Side Effects
Sodium) Potassium) BENZOATE Calcium)	Anti-bacterial Anti-fungal	Asthma, skin rashes, numbness of mouth, known aspirin sensitivity
Potassium metabisulphite and sulphites	Preservative in fruit, wine, beer: stops fermentation.	Asthma, skin rashes, abdominal bloating, excess gas. May reduce Vitamin B_1 in food.
Potassium nitrate (saltpetre)	Food preservative especially of meats. Protects *very effectively* against toxic bacteria in meats.	Severe abdominal pain and cramps muscle weakness, irregular heart action.
Sulphur dioxide	Preservative Bleaching agent. Vitamin C stabilizer.	Vitamin E reduced in flour after being bleached. Gas, indigestion, diarrhoea.

Table 15

Other harmful colouring agents are red, blue and green dyes, often used in sweets, pastries, carbonated drinks, fruit juices, ice cream, maraschino cherries, jellies, hot dogs, convenience foods, pickles and chewing gums.

Preservatives may be natural, such as vinegar, salt and sulphur. The addition to food of certain herbs may also have a preservative effect. Other preservatives have to be used with great care, and only when preservation of food is necessary because it cannot be eaten fresh.

Such preservatives are found in prawns, confectionery, margarine, fruit pies, soft drinks, salad dressings, barbecue sauces, soya sauce, pickled onions, cabbage, Camden tablets used in preserving fruit and home-made wine, cider, beer, cooked meats, sausages, cured meat products, bacon, ham and many products sold at delicatessen counters.

Antioxidants prevent oxygen from turning oils and fats rancid. Many prepackaged foods contain them. Some natural substances such as vitamin C and E fulfil the same purpose. For example, vitamin C in fruit prevents oxygenation, reducing the browning that may occur with exposure to air. It is also a colour preservative. Vitamin E, occurring either naturally or synthetically, reduces the rancidity that may result in oils exposed to air.

Potentially Harmful Antioxidants

Substance	Action	Possible Side Effects
Propyl gallate	Antioxidant for oils and fats	Gastric irritation, asthma, possible liver damage and reproductive problems
Butylated hydroxyanisole (BHA)	Antioxidant for oils and fats	Raises cholesterol blood levels
Butylated hydroxytoluene (BHT)	Prevents flavour deterioration	Reduces Vitamin D; causes blood cell changes, behavioural problems

Table 16

Antioxidants are found in beverages, ice cream , diced fruits, potato crisps, chewing gum, some breakfast cereals, some packaging materials using plastic film, rubber gaskets in food-jar sealers, enriched savoury rice, Scotch eggs, cheese spread, salted peanuts, sachet marinades and dehydrated mashed potatoes.

Total bans on the use of BHT and possibly BHA, both popular antioxidants, are being considered in Europe, Scandinavia and Australia.

Potentially Harmful Solvents

Substance	Action	Possible Side Effects
Glycerol	Solvent; food sweetener	Headache, thirst, alterations in blood sugar levels

Table 17

Solvents are used in liqueur chocolates, confectionery and in the icings for cakes.

Emulsifiers are found in chocolate, soft margarines, vermicelli, yoghurt whips and dessert mixes. Stabilizing Irish moss (carageenan), can be found in such products as ice cream, milk shakes, desserts, cheese, quick-setting jelly mix, blancmanges, salad dressings and sour cream. Products containing polyphosphates may include cheese, frozen turkey, meat loaf, frozen fish fingers, fish cakes, meat and ham loaf, and canned sausages.

Potentially Harmful Emulsifiers and Stabilizers

Substance	Action	Possible Side Effects
Calcium disodium EDTA	Chelating substance and stabilizer	Vomiting, diarrhoea, abdominal cramps. May reduce absorption of iron, zinc and copper.
Phosphates and poly-phosphates	Emulsifier and texturizer	Possible digestive problems and enzyme reduction.

Table 18

Most *emulsifiers* are quite safe and naturally occurring, such as lecithin, as found in soya beans and egg yolks. These products reduce the thickness of a substance. *Stabilizers* often thicken products, usually by causing gelling and bulking. A common stabilizer is carboxymethylcellulose. *Polyphosphates* are very hydrophilic; they attract water, increasing the weight of the product in which they are used. Some products can have their weight increased by as much as 40 per cent and of course the price will rise correspondingly, even though the weight gain is only in water.

Finally, a few words about *monosodium glutamate* (MSG), which is probably one of the most talked about additives. MSG occurs naturally as a Japanese seaweed, Seatango. It can also be prepared from wheat gluten and sugar beet. Its main use is as a flavour enhancer of protein food — it either stimulates the taste buds or increases saliva production. It is used extensively in Chinese restaurants, giving rise to 'Chinese restaurant syndrome', some of whose symptoms are headache, asthma, heart palpitations, nausea and muscle weakness. Migraine attacks have also been reported. MSG is commonly found in heat-and-serve convenience foods, meats, stews, meat tenderizers, canned and frozen vegetables, most canned soups and soup mixes, condiments and seasonings, potato crisps and flavoured noodles.

Check the labels first. MSG content is not always consistent. For example, a Pea Soup may contain MSG while the same company's Green Pea Soup may not. One company's Chicken Nuggets may contain MSG, while another convenience chicken product made by the same company may not.

If you suffer or suspect you suffer, from PMS symptoms, it is most important that you become aware, as all consumers should, of the additives in your food. It is evident that some are required and are beneficial to food preservation, while others are highly questionable and some hazardous. Certain additives may, in your case, be aggravating PMS symptoms. Read the label on the foods you buy. Be informed.

Epilogue

Looking Ahead

As research proceeds, Pre-Menstrual Syndrome will very probably emerge as being the end result of a defective chain of events, each link in the chain being a connecting biochemical process, the start of which may well be influenced by a hereditary factor. If all the links in the chain are strong, there will be no PMS. Strengthening these links in logical sequence, according to the ten-point key regime of the treatment, lays the ground-work for the formation and proper balance of prostaglandins and hormones such as progesterone. Correction and prevention of PMS follows.

Current research into early links in the chain focusses on the pineal gland and the hypothalamus. It is here that the so-called neurotransmitters of total control are housed. The complex peptides alpha-MSH (melanocyte stimulating hormones) and beta-endorphin from the hypothalamus, after their release into the cerebrospinal fluid, may provide the all-important link in the chain. But until these initiating factors are understood, the symptoms resulting from their defectiveness can be repaired by the treatment programme outlined in this book, maintaining the prostaglandins in balance and supplying extra progesterone as needed to satisfy and fill the progesterone receptors on cell surfaces.

In the early 1970s, shortly after the CAT scan (computerized axial tomography X-ray scanner) opened up new vistas of medical diagnosis, Nuclear Magnetic Imaging (NMI) was born. This sophisticated, non-invasive technique produces superb images of organs protected by bone and cartilage such as the brain, the nervous system and the pelvic organs — especially of women. Even newer is Positron Emission Tomography (PET).

Secondly, PET has the ability to assess the chemical composition of tissue. This has enormous possibilities as far as illness is concerned because, within the next few years, it will be possible to diagnose accurately the cause of a deficiency disease or to determine which body chemical is present in excess and where it is located. Perhaps PET will be able to indicate where the abnormal or defective links in the chain of PMS are. The strengthening or repair of those links through appropriate treatment will then be possible.

The increasing interest many women have shown in Pre-Menstrual Syndrome during the last few years has caused some concern and confusion amongst feminist groups. Some have been reluctant to even accept the existence of PMS; others tacitly acknowledge that it is there; others prefer to define it simply as a 'woman's problem'. Surely a denial of its existence and a referral to it as a female problem creates a feeling of inferiority in some women towards other women and towards men. Some fear that equal rights might be compromised, that the stigma of PMS would make a woman less capable and responsible in the workforce.

It is debatable whether court cases in which PMS is used as the defence assist or damage women's equal rights. When a sentence is reduced on the grounds of 'diminished responsibility', then it is logical that such a phrase could quite easily and readily be applied to others who have committed no crime but may have similar symptoms. How wrong this would be and how small the minds of those who would, or could, draw such a parallel. If it is fully recognized and understood that PMS is a physical internal disorder, a medical problem that can be treated and corrected, then it becomes like any other physical problem. It should be treated openly, with skill, understanding and humanity. It is wrong for society, or any group in society, to use a correctable medical problem as an excuse for denying women equal rights in the workforce.

Today, competition is all-important; modern women are showing that they can aspire to and hold, equally with men, the highest offices in government, in professions, in business and even in the exploration of outer space. To compete and to accomplish, physical and emotional fitness is essential. Women who have had PMS diagnosed and corrected have a feeling of well-being that results in a greater enjoyment of a full and active life. They have a feeling of freedom, month after month after month.

Appendix A

Allergy Food Lists and Food Families
Diets Without Wheat _____ Foods to Avoid

Beverages
Beer; Malted Chocolate Drink; coffee substitutes; instant coffee unless 100 per cent coffee; gin; malted milk; whisky.

Breads, crackers and rolls
All breads including pumpernickel, rye, oatmeal and corn; scones; crackers; gluten bread; pancakes; hot breads and rolls; pretzels; rusks; waffles.

Cereals
All-Bran, Bran Flakes; Cheerios; Semolina; muesli type; Grapenuts; Grape-nut flakes; Ready Brek; Puffed Wheat; Shredded Wheat; Special K; Wheat Flakes; wheatgerm; Weetos.

Desserts
Cakes or biscuits (homemade, from mixes, or bakery); doughnuts; ice cream; ice cream cones; pies; puddings.

Flour
All-purpose; brown wheat flour; white; wholemeal

Gravies and sauces
Any thickened with flour.

Meats
Canned meat dishes such as stews; chilli; frankfurters, luncheon meats or sausage in which wheat has been used as a filler; meats prepared with bread, rusk or flour, such as croquettes and meat loaf; stews thickened with flour or made with dumplings; stuffings and commercial stuffing mixes.

Pasta
Macaroni; noodles; spaghetti; etc.

Salad dressings
Any thickened with flour.

Soups
Bouillon cubes; commercial; canned.

NOTE: Quick breads can be made from rice, potato, rye or

other flours, but adjustments in baking temperature and time must be made. The amount of baking powder is increased because of the lack of gluten in these flours. The finished products differ in texture from those prepared from wheat. They should be stored in the freezer rather than in the refrigerator, because they tend to dry out quickly.

Diets Without Corn _____ Foods to Avoid

Beverages
Ale; beer; carbonated; coffee lighteners; grape juice; instant tea; milk substitutes; soya milks; whisky.

Breads, crackers and rolls
Corn breads or rolls; muffins; digestive biscuits.

Cereals
Cornmeal; hominy; Corn Flakes; Grapenuts.

Desserts
Cakes; candied fruits; canned or frozen fruit or juices; cream pies; ice cream; pastries; pudding mixes; sherbet.

Fats
Corn oil; corn oil margarine; gravies and salad dressings thickened with cornflour; mayonnaise, salad dressings and shortenings unless the source of oil is specified.

Flours and thickeners
Cornmeal; cornflour.

Meats
Bacon; hams (cured, tenderized); luncheon meats; sausage.

Soups
All commercial; homemade thickened with cornflour.

Sweet foods
All sweets; cane sugar; corn syrups; corn sugars; corn-based maple syrups; artificial vanilla; jams, jellies, preserves.

Vegetables
Beets; corn on the cob; mixed vegetables containing corn; canned sweetcorn.

Miscellaneous
Baking powders; batters for frying; ketchup; chewing gum; cheese spreads; Chinese foods; commercial baking, cake, pancake, pastry and pudding mixes; confectioner's sugar; distilled vinegar; monosodium glutamate; peanut butter; popcorn; sandwich spreads; sauces; toppings; vitamin capsules; yeast.

Diets Without Milk ——————— Foods to Avoid

Milk
All forms; buttermilk, evaporated, fresh whole or skimmed; malted; yoghurt.

Beverages
Chocolate; cocoa; Chocolate Malted Drink; Ovaltine.

Breads and rolls
Any made with milk (most breads contain milk); bread mixes; pancakes; soda crackers; waffles.

Cereals
Cream of rice; Instant Semolina; Special K.

Cheese
All kinds; cheese dips and spreads.

Desserts
Cakes; biscuits; custard; doughnuts; ice cream; mixes of all types; pastry made with butter or margarine; pies with cream fillings such as chocolate, coconut, cream, custard, lemon; puddings with milk; sherbet.

Fats
Butter; cream; margarine.

Meats
Frankfurters; luncheon meats; meat loaf — unless 100 per cent meat.

Sauces
Any made with butter, margarine, milk or cream.

Soups
Bisques; chowders; cream.

Sweets
Caramels; chocolate toffees.

Vegetables
Served au gratin; mashed potatoes; any seasoned with butter or margarine; scalloped; any with cream sauce.

Food Families

Family	Other Members
Apple	Apple, pear, quince, pectin
Arrowroot	Arrowroot
Banana	Banana, plantain
Beech	Chestnut

Birch	Filbert, hazelnut
Bird	Chicken and eggs, duck and eggs, turkey, goose, pheasant, grouse
Bovine	Beef, veal, cow's milk, butter, cream cheese, gelatine, yoghurt, whey
Brazil	Brazil nuts
Buckwheat	Buckwheat, rhubarb, garden sorrel
Cactus	Tequila
Cashew	Cashew nuts, pistachios, mangoes
Cereal	Corn, cornmeal, cornflour, corn oil, corn syrup, dextrose, glucose
	Wheat, wheat flour
	Rye, oats, barley, malt, rice, sorghum, millet
	Cane sugar, molasses, bamboo shoots
	Gluten-free flours, bran, semolina
Chicory	Chicory
Chocolate	Cocoa, chocolate, cola
Citrus	Lemon, orange, grapefruit, lime, tangerine, satsuma, citron peel, angostura (bitters)
Composite	Lettuce, endive, artichoke, dandelion, sunflower, sesame, safflower, camomile, absinthe, vermouth
Crustacean	Crab, crayfish, lobster, shrimp, prawn
Fish, freshwater	Sturgeon, salmon, bass, perch, trout
Fish, saltwater	Herring, anchovy, cod, sea bass, sea trout, mackerel, tuna, flounder, sole, swordfish
Fungi	Mushroom, yeast, antibiotics
Game	Venison, rabbit
Ginger	Ginger, turmeric
Goat	Goats milk and cheese
Gooseberry	Gooseberry, currants
Gourd	Cucumber, melon, pumpkin (marrow) courgette, cantaloupe, acorn squash
Grape	Grape, raisin, sultana, cream of tartar, tartaric acid, wine, wine vinegar, brandy, champagne
Heath	Cranberry, blueberry, bilberry
Honey	Honey
Iris	Saffron

Laurel	Avocado, cinnamon, bay leaf, sassafras root
Legumes	Peas, beans, soya beans, lentils, peanuts, liquorice, gum tragacanth
Lily	Onion, garlic, asparagus, chives, leeks
Madder	Coffee
Mint	Peppermint, spearmint, basil, rosemary, marjoram, sage, thyme, Chinese artichoke
Morning glory	Sweet potato
Mulberry	Mulberry, fig, hop, breadfruit
Mustard	Mustard, cabbage, cauliflower, broccoli, swede, Brussels sprouts, turnip, kale, radish, horseradish, watercress
Myrtle	Guava, allspice, clove
Nutmeg	Nutmeg, mace
Olive	Black and green olives, olive oil, stuffed olives
Orchid	Vanilla
Palm	Coconut, date, sago
Papaya	Papaya, papain
Parsley	Carrots, parsnips, celery, parsley, anise, caraway dill, fennel, angelica, cumin, celeriac
Pepper	Black and white pepper, peppercorn
Pig	Pork, bacon, ham
Pine	Juniper, pine nut
Pineapple	Pineapple
Plum	Plum, almond, peach, apricot, cherries, prunes, nectarines
Pomegranate	Pomegranate
Poppy	Poppy seed
Potato	Potato, tomato, aubergine, paprika, cayenne pepper, chilli, sweet pepper
Seafood	Abalone, clam, mussel, oyster, scallop, squid
Sheep	Lamb and mutton
Tea	Tea
Walnut	Walnut, hickory nut, butternut
Water chestnut	Chinese water chestnuts
Yam	Yam

Appendix B

Low Sodium Recipes

Hearty Lentil Soup	Metric	Imperial
Stock/water	1.5 l	2½ pt
Safflower oil	15 ml	1 tbsp
Carrots (medium), chopped	3	3
Leeks (medium), sliced	2	2
Onion (medium), chopped	1	1
Tomatoes (medium) OR	450 g	1 lb
no-salt-added canned plum		
tomatoes	450 ml	¾ pt
Red lentils	450 g	1 lb
Bouquet garni*		
Ground cumin (optional)	15 ml	1 tbsp
Parsley, chopped	15 ml	1 tbsp

1. Fry the carrots, leeks, and onion in the oil to which you have added 30–45ml/2–3 tbsp. of stock/water.
2. Chop the tomatoes and add them to the vegetables. Add lentils, bouquet garni and cumin. Pour on the remaining stock/water.
   N.B. If using canned tomatoes, add the tomatoes and the juice together with the lentils, but decrease the amount of stock/water by 100 ml/4fl oz.
3. Bring all ingredients to a boil, then lower the heat and simmer for approximately 1½ hours.
4. Remove bouquet garni and serve piping hot, garnished with parsley.

Serves 6. 46 mg sodium approx. per serving.

*Bouquet garni is a mixture of crushed parsley stalks, peppercorns, and a slice of onion, wrapped in muslin and tied.

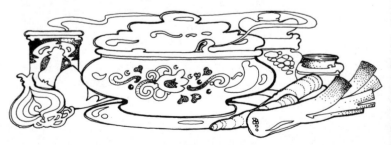

Paprika Bean Soup	Metric	Imperial
Safflower oil	30 ml	2 tbsp
Onions (medium), peeled and sliced	2	2
Paprika	30 ml	2 tbsp
Red peppers (medium), cored, and seeds removed, cut into strips	2	2
Canned plum tomatoes (no salt added)	775 ml	1¼ pt
Stock/water	500 ml	¾ pt
Haricot beans (soaked overnight and partially cooked)	175 g	6 oz
Pinto beans (soaked overnight and partially cooked)	175 g	6 oz
Red kidney beans (soaked overnight and partially cooked)	175 g	6 oz

1. Heat the oil in a pan, and add the onions. Sauté until soft and translucent. Add the paprika, and cook for a few minutes.
2. Add the sliced red peppers and can of plum tomatoes. Bring to a boil and then simmer for 20 minutes.
3. Pour on the stock/water. Add the beans to the pan and continue cooking for 20–30 minutes, until beans are cooked.
4. Serve with a spoonful of skimmed milk yoghurt, if desired.

Serves 4. 25 mg sodium approx. per serving, without the yoghurt.

Split Pea Chowder	Metric	Imperial
Yellow split peas (soaked overnight)	225 g	8 oz
Leeks (medium), cleaned and sliced	2	2
Carrots (medium), peeled and diced	2	2
Onion (medium), chopped	1	1
Stock/water	1.25 l	2 pt
Black pepper to taste		
Potatoes, scrubbed and sliced	500 g	1 lb

1. Wash the soaked split peas and place in a saucepan together with the leeks, carrots and onion.
2. Pour the stock/water over the vegetables, bring to the boil, and simmer for 30–40 minutes.
3. Season the soup with pepper and add the sliced potatoes; cook for a further 30 minutes.
4. Serve hot with wholemeal rolls.

Serves 4. 35mg sodium approx. per serving.

Chicken Vegetable Soup

Chicken Vegetable Soup	Metric	Imperial
Pinto beans or haricot beans (soaked overnight and partially cooked)	175 g	6 oz
Dried peas/Marrowfat peas (soaked and partially cooked)	175 g	6 oz
Chicken breasts, skinned	300 g	10 oz
Onion (medium), sliced	1	1
Carrot (large), cut into strips	1	1
Leeks (medium), cut into strips	2	2
Bouquet garni		
Peppercorns	6	6
Water	1.5 l	2½ pt
Courgette (medium), cut into strips	1	1
Black pepper to taste		

1. Place the partially cooked beans and peas, chicken breast, onion, carrot and leeks in a saucepan together with the bouquet garni and 6 black peppercorns. Pour on the water, bring to the boil and simmer for 30 minutes or until chicken is cooked.
2. Remove chicken, bouquet garni and peppercorns from saucepan. Take the chicken flesh from the bone and cut into strips. Return to saucepan together with courgettes, and cook, covered, for 10 minutes. Adjust pepper seasoning.
3. Serve with crusty bread.

Serves 4. 60 mg sodium approx. per serving.

Cabbage, Potato and Tomato Salad

Cabbage, Potato and Tomato Salad	Metric	Imperial
White or firm green cabbage* (small), finely shredded	700 g	1½ lb
Safflower oil	125 ml	7 tbsp
Black pepper to taste		
Wine vinegar	30 ml	2 tbsp
Bunch of spring onions, sliced	1	1
New potatoes or old potatoes**	375 g	12 oz.
Mustard powder	5 ml	1 tsp
Ripe, firm tomatoes, sliced	500 g	1 lb
Mixed herbs, finely chopped	15–30 ml	1–2 tbsp

1. Coat the shredded cabbage with 60 ml oil/4 tbsp. Season with black pepper and 15 ml/1 tbsp wine vinegar, and add the sliced spring onions. Cover and refrigerate for 30 minutes.
2. Cook the potatoes in their skins. Slice while still hot and mix with a dressing made with the mustard, remaining oil, wine vinegar and black pepper.
3. Mix the potatoes with the cabbage and place in a bowl. Edge the bowl with sliced tomatoes and garnish with finely chopped mixed herbs.

*Use red and green cabbage in equal quantities for a more colourful combination.
**If using old potatoes, choose a floury variety that will produce a dry texture when cooked.
Serves 6–9. 25 mg sodium approx. per serving.

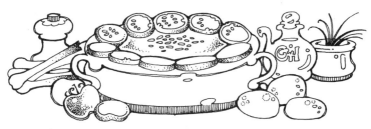

Salad Niçoise	**Metric**	**Imperial**
Crisp lettuce, shredded and torn	1	1
Tuna (packed in water) OR shredded cooked breast of chicken	175 g	6 oz
Mixed herbs, chopped	30 ml	2 tbsp
Green beans OR mange tout, cooked	175 g	6 oz
Ripe, firm tomatoes, sliced (approx. 1 lb/500 g)	4	4
Cucumber, sliced or diced	½	½
French dressing		
Eggs (large), hardboiled and quartered	2	2

1. Place layer of lettuce on the bottom of a bowl or dish. Flake the tuna. Layer the ingredients as follows: tuna or chicken, 15 ml chopped herbs, green beans or mange tout, sliced tomatoes, sliced or diced cucumber and remaining herbs.
2. Toss all ingredients with French dressing and garnish with quarters of hardboiled egg.

French Dressing	Metric	Imperial
Safflower oil	45 ml	3 tbsp
Freshly ground black pepper to taste		
Dry mustard	pinch	pinch
Wine vinegar	15 ml	1 tbsp

1. Mix oil and seasonings, then add vinegar and mix well.
   N.B. If making a larger quantity, place all ingredients in a bottle or jar and shake well.

For 4 using tuna _____ 86 mg sodium approx. per serving.
For 6 using tuna _____ 50 mg sodium approx. per serving.
For 4 using chicken ___ 83 mg sodium approx. per serving.
For 6 using chicken ___ 56 mg sodium approx. per serving.

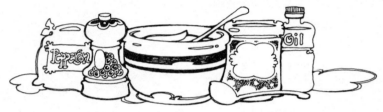

Tabouli	Metric	Imperial
Burghul (cracked wheat)	175 g	6 oz
Firm, ripe tomatoes (medium)	2	2
Red pepper (medium), chopped	1	1
Green pepper (medium), chopped	1	1
Bunch of spring onions, chopped	1	1
Safflower oil	45 ml	3 tbsp
Freshly ground black pepper to taste		
Fresh mint, chopped	10 ml	2 tsp
Fresh parsley, chopped	15 ml	1 tbsp
Lemon juice	45 ml	3 tbsp

1. Soak the burghul wheat in cold water for 1 hour. Drain and wrap in a clean tea towel; squeeze out the moisture.
2. Skin tomatoes, cut into quarters, remove and discard seeds and shred tomato flesh.
3. Core and seed the peppers, then chop finely.
4. Finely chop spring onions.
5. Mix all ingredients together. Season to taste.

Serves 4. 8 mg sodium approx. per serving.

Prawn and Tomato Filled Courgettes	Metric	Imperial
Courgettes (6 in./24 cm long)	2	2
Shallot, finely chopped	1	1
Carrot (small), finely diced	1	1
Safflower oil	20 ml	4 tsp
Paprika	5 ml	1 tsp
No-salt-added canned plum tomatoes	450 ml	¾ pt
Bouquet garni		
Prawns, canned, well washed in fine sieve	115 g	4½ oz
Wholemeal breadcrumbs	30 ml	2 tbsp

1. Preheat oven to 180°C/350°F/Gas Mark 4. Remove courgette ends and halve lengthwise, but do not peel. Scoop out the seedy flesh in the centre, using a teaspoon or melon baller. Steam the courgette halves for 3–5 minutes or until tender but crisp. Drain well and arrange in an oiled baking dish.
2. Soften chopped shallot and diced carrot in the safflower oil over medium heat. Add paprika and cook for a few minutes, then add tomatoes and simmer for 30–45 minutes with the bouquet garni, until mixture forms a thick pulp.
3. Remove bouquet garni from tomato pulp. Add the well washed and drained prawns; mix well. Pile filling into courgette cases. Sprinkle with breadcrumbs, and bake for 20–30 minutes, until hot.

Serves 2 as a main course or 4 as an accompaniment or snack.

As a main course, 114 mg sodium approx. per person.
As an accompaniment, 57 mg sodium approx. per person.

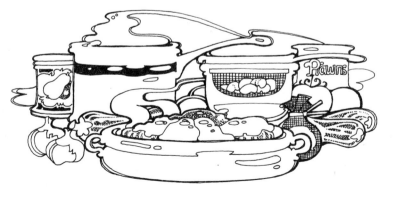

Fish Gratin	Metric	Imperial
White fish (sole, haddock or flounder)	375 g	12 oz
Skimmed milk	300 ml	½ pt
Bouquet garni		
Safflower oil	30 ml	2 tbsp
Mushrooms, sliced	125 g	4 oz
Unbleached flour	30 ml	2 tbsp
Skimmed milk, from poaching fish	300 ml	½ pt
Tomatoes (medium), skinned, seeded and quartered	3	3
Mashed potatoes (freshly boiled in skins, then peeled and sieved, seasoned with pepper and grated nutmeg)	500 g	1 lb

1. Poach fish in the skimmed milk with the bouquet garni until it flakes easily. Cool, strain the milk (reserving it) and flake the fish.
2. *Sauce*: Heat oil in a pan. Fry sliced mushrooms briskly for 2–3 minutes, then blend in flour. Remove from heat and add liquid from the poached fish, stirring until thickened. Add fish and tomato quarters that have been cut in three.
3. In a fireproof, oiled dish make a border of mashed potato and into the centre pour the fish mixture. Brown under a hot grill.

Serves 4. 120 mg sodium approx. per serving.

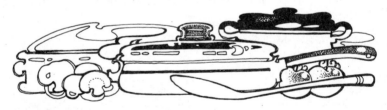

Chicken Breasts with Mushroom Stuffing	Metric	Imperial
Shallot, finely chopped	1	1
Safflower oil	15 ml	1 tbsp
Mushrooms, chopped	125 g	4 oz
Fresh whole-meal breadcrumbs	30 ml	2 tbsp
Mixed chopped herbs	30 ml	2 tbsp
Egg white, slightly beaten	15 ml	1 tbsp
Boneless skinned chicken breasts, approx. 4 oz/125 g each	4	4
Chicken stock OR dry white wine	60 ml	4 tbsp

1. Preheat oven to 180°C/350°F/Gas Mark 4. Soften shallot in oil. Add mushrooms and fry briskly for a few minutes. Cool mushroom and shallot mixture, then add breadcrumbs and herbs. Mix in egg white to bind mixture.
2. Flatten chicken breasts with a rolling pin. Place two together with half the stuffing between them. Tie with kitchen string. Repeat with the other two breasts.
3. Place chicken breasts on oiled circles of foil. Sprinkle with chicken stock or white wine, and then seal.
4. Place the two packages on a grid over a pan of warm water and cook in the oven for 30–40 minutes, until tender.
5. Serve either hot or cold, sliced.

Serves 4. 120 mg of sodium approx. per serving.

Chicken with Tangy Tomato Sauce	**Metric**	**Imperial**
Chicken breasts, boneless and skinned, approx. 4 oz/125g each	4	4
No salt added canned plum tomatoes	500 ml	¾ pt
Black peppercorns	12	12
Red wine vinegar	50 ml	2 fl oz
Chicken stock	225 ml	8 fl oz
Marjoram, chopped	5 ml	1 tsp
Bayleaf	1	1
Potato flour, for thickening.		

1. Heat a non-stick frying pan over medium heat and brown chicken breasts on both sides, about 2 minutes. Remove chicken breasts and place on a rack to cool.
2. In a pan place the tomatoes, peppercorns and vinegar, and bring to the boil and cook for 10 minutes. Add chicken stock, marjoram and bayleaf; reduce heat and simmer for a further 10 minutes.
3. Place the cooled chicken in a casserole and pour over the tomato sauce. Simmer for about 20 minutes until chicken is tender.
4. Pour tomato sauce from casserole into a pan and simmer until reduced to about 300 ml. Pass sauce through a sieve and season with freshly ground black pepper, if required. If the sauce is too thin, thicken with a little potato flour.
5. Spoon sauce over chicken in the casserole and reheat. Serve with brown basmati rice.

Serves 4. 78 mg sodium approx. per serving without rice.

Stuffed Peppers	Metric	Imperial
Peppers (red, green, yellow)	4	4
Brown basmati rice	125 g	4 oz
Onion, finely chopped	1	1
Mushrooms, sliced	125 g	4 oz
Chicken breast, cooked and diced	125 g	4 oz
Safflower oil	30–45 ml	2–3 tbsp
Chicken stock*	300 ml	½ pt
Mixed herbs, chopped	30 ml	2 tbsp

1. Wash and drain basmati rice; dry thoroughly.
2. Preheat oven to 180°C/350°F/Gas Mark 4. Remove tops, core and seeds of peppers. Steam for 10 minutes. Refresh under cold water to set colour.
3. Over medium heat soften onion in the oil. Add mushrooms and increase heat to drive off excess moisture. Add rice and cook for 5–10 minutes. Add stock to pan and cover rice well, cook over medium heat until rice is tender. Stir in diced cooked chicken and herbs to cooled mixture.
4. Pile rice mixture into peppers, and place in a dish with 1.5 cm/½ inch of water. Bake peppers until tender, about 30–45 minutes.
5. Serve with tomato sauce.

Alternative: use all red peppers and prawns instead of chicken in filling.
Serves 4 — 50 mg sodium approx. per serving without sauce, using chicken.

* If you have no chicken stock use a low salt vegetable bouillon cube.

Ratatouille	Metric	Imperial
Safflower oil	5 ml	1 tsp
Onion (medium), sliced	1	1
Green pepper (medium), sliced	1	1
Red pepper (medium), sliced	1	1
Courgette (medium), sliced	3	3
Canned plum tomatoes, no salt added, chopped with juice OR	450 ml	¾ pt
Fresh tomatoes, skinned, seeded and chopped	700 g	1½ lb
Black pepper to taste		
Marjoram or basil	pinch	pinch

1. Preheat oven to 190°C/375°F/Gas Mark 5. Brush ovenproof casserole with safflower oil.
2. Place onion, peppers and courgette in the casserole. Add black pepper, herbs and tomatoes including the juice.
3. Bake for 30–45 minutes or until vegetables are tender but not soft.
4. Serve hot or cold.

Serves 4. 22 mg sodium approx. per serving

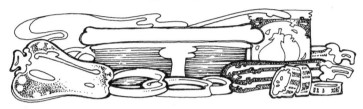

Brown Basmati Rice
Allow 50 g/2 oz rice per person.

1. Soak rice in cold water for about 1 hour to remove excess starch.
2. Drain well and rinse under cold water. Place rice in a saucepan and cover with cold water. Bring to the boil and simmer until rice is tender and water absorbed, 5–10 minutes.

2 mg sodium approx. per serving.

Tomato Sauce	Metric	Imperial
Safflower oil	30 ml	2 tbsp
Onion (medium), chopped finely	1	1
Carrot (medium), chopped finely	1	1
Canned plum tomatoes (no salt added)	775 ml	1¼ pt
Bay leaf	1	1
Black pepper to taste		
Chopped mixed herbs (optional)		

1. Heat oil over medium heat and soften onion and carrot.
2. Add canned tomatoes and bay leaf and bring to the boil. Then simmer until mixture is reduced to a thickish pulp.
3. Cool tomatoes; liquidize and sieve to remove seeds. Return tomato liquid to rinsed-out pan and reduce over heat if sauce is still too thin. Add pepper and herbs when liquidized.

75 mg sodium approx.

Appendix C

Low Sugar/Low Sodium Recipes

Baked Apple with Raisins and Walnuts

	Metric	Imperial
Apples (Newtons or Granny Smiths)	4	4
Sultanas	50 g	2 oz
Walnuts, coarsely chopped	25 g	1 oz

1. Preheat oven to 350°F/180°C/Gas Mark 4. Core apples and stuff with a mixture of sultanas and chopped walnuts. Place in a shallow pie dish which contains ¼ in/1 cm water. Bake for 30 minutes or until cooked.
2. Serve warm, garnished with a spoonful of skimmed milk yoghurt if desired.

Serves 4. 8 mg sodium approx. per serving, without the yoghurt.

Wholemeal Pancakes

	Metric	Imperial
Wholemeal flour	75 g	3 oz
Unbleached plain flour	25 g	1 oz
Egg (large)	1	1
Skimmed milk	350 ml	12 fl oz
Safflower oil, a little		

1. Place flours into a bowl and add the egg and skimmed milk. Beat well. Allow to stand 10 minutes.
2. Wipe nonstick frying pan with a little oil and then heat over medium heat. Pour batter into the pan, allowing it to cover the base of the pan as thinly as possible. Cook approximately 1 minute; then toss and cook the other side.
3. Between pancakes you may need to wipe the pan with a little oil.
4. Serve immediately, or pile the pancakes with greaseproof paper between them.
5. Serving suggestion: place a spoonful of part-skimmed ricotta cheese on pancake, fold over, and top with a spoonful of fruit purée or fruit sauce. Place under a hot grill to heat through before serving.

Makes 12. 22 mg sodium approx. per pancake, without cheese or fruit purée.

Fruit Crisp	Metric	Imperial
Apples/rhubarb/pears	500 g	1 lb
Orange (large), juice	1	1
Wholemeal flour	50 g	2 oz
Coarse oatmeal	25 g	1 oz
Low sodium margarine	50 g	2 oz
Walnuts, chopped	25 g	1 oz

1. Preheat oven to 400°F/200°C/Gas Mark 6. Place prepared fruit (sliced apples or pears, or chopped rhubarb) in a deep pie dish. Pour orange juice over fruit.
2. In a bowl, sift flour, add oatmeal, and then rub in margarine until mixture is like breadcrumbs, but not oily. Stir in chopped walnuts.
3. Sprinkle evenly over fruit. Place high in oven and bake for 20 minutes or until the top is crunchy and lightly browned.

Serves 4. 6 mg sodium approx. per serving.

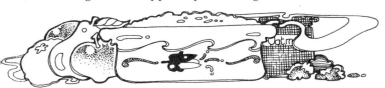

Wholemeal Almond Scones	Metric	Imperial
Wholemeal flour	125 g	4 oz
Plain flour	50 g	2 oz
Low sodium baking powder	30 ml	6 tsp
Low sodium margarine	50 g	2 oz
Ground almonds	50 g	2 oz
Skimmed milk	50–100 ml	2–4 fl oz
Sultanas (optional)	50 g	2 oz

1. Preheat oven to 425°F/220°C/Gas Mark 7. Place whole-meal flour in a bowl, sift in cake and pastry flour and low sodium baking powder.
2. Rub in margarine until like fine breadcrumbs. Mix in ground almonds. Add sultanas. Add skimmed milk and mix all ingredients to a soft dough.
3. Knead dough lightly on a floured surface. Roll out to 2 cm/¾ in thickness, cut into rounds and place on a floured baking tray.
4. Bake scones for approximately 15 minutes, or until golden brown.

Makes 6. 14 mg sodium approx. per scone.

Seven Grain Cereal Wholemeal Bread	Metric	Imperial
Wholemeal flour	350 g	12 oz
Seven grain cereal mix OR muesli base	50 g	2 oz
Unbleached plain flour	125 g	4 oz
Skimmed milk	225 ml	8 fl oz
Safflower oil	50ml	2 fl oz
Warm water	50 ml	2 fl oz
Sugar	pinch	pinch
Dried yeast	10 ml	2 tsp

1. Warm a mixing bowl and place wholemeal flour and seven grain cereal mix or muesli base in bowl. Sift flour into bowl.
2. Warm milk and oil. In a small bowl dissolve sugar in hand-warm water. Sprinkle yeast over water and set aside until frothy on top.
3. Make a well in the centre of dry ingredients, and to this add the frothy yeast liquid and the milk and oil, and mix to a dough.
4. Turn dough out onto a floured board and knead for 10 minutes to develop the gluten.
5. Place dough into an oiled bowl or plastic bag and leave in a warm place to double in size.
6. Preheat oven to 425°F/220°C/Gas Mark 7. Oil tins or baking trays.
7. Turn out dough when risen and knead for a couple of minutes before dividing into 2 loaves or 12 rolls. Shape dough for loaves or rolls and place in oiled tins or baking tray in a plastic bag and leave to double in size.
8. When doubled in size, bake rolls for 20 minutes or loaves for 30 minutes or until done.
9. To test that bread or rolls are done, tap the bottom. If it sounds hollow, it is ready.
10. Allow bread to cool on a rack.

Makes 2 loaves or 12 rolls. 15 mg sodium approx. per roll.

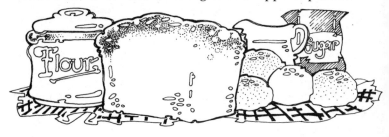

Oatcakes

	Metric	Imperial
Low sodium margarine	25 g	1 oz
Water	100 ml	4 fl oz
Medium oatmeal	225 g	8 oz
Low sodium baking powder	pinch	pinch

1. Preheat oven to 180°C/350°F/Gas Mark 4. Melt margarine in water over low heat.
2. In a bowl, stir together oatmeal and low sodium baking powder. Add melted margarine and water mixture. Mix to a stiff dough.
3. Knead dough lightly on a floured surface, then roll out thinly and cut into 4 cm/1½ in rounds. Place on a baking sheet and bake for 20–30 minutes or until crisp.

Makes 16. 5 mg sodium approx. per oatcake.

Cranberry and Apple Oaties

	Metric	Imperial
Low sodium margarine	125 g	4 oz
Juice and grated rind of orange (large)	1	1
Rolled oats	125 g	4 oz
Wholemeal flour	125 g	4 oz
Cranberries, frozen	225 g	8 oz
Apples (Newton or Granny Smiths), peeled, cored and sliced	300 g	12 oz
Walnuts, chopped	50 g	2 oz

1. Preheat oven to 180°C/350°F/Gas Mark 4. Oil an 18-cm/7-in square shallow tin.
2. Melt margarine, add half the orange juice, the rolled oats and whole-meal flour. Stir well.
3. Press half the oat mixture into base of tin.
4. In a separate pan, place cranberries, remaining orange juice made up to 50 ml/2 fl oz with water, and grated orange rind. Bring to the boil and then simmer for a few minutes. Add prepared apples and cook with cranberries. When a thick pulp, remove from heat and allow to cool.
5. Place cranberry/apple mixture on top of oat base. Sprinkle with walnuts and remaining oat mixture. Bake in the centre of the oven until golden brown, about 25 minutes.
6. Cut into slices while in the tin and leave to cool.

Makes 8 slices. 5 mg sodium approx. per slice.

Orange Carrot Cake

	Metric	Imperial
Wholemeal flour	175 g	6 oz
Unbleached plain flour	125 g	4 oz
Low sodium baking powder	20 ml	4 tsp
Fructose	15 ml	1 tbsp
Ground almonds	30 ml	2 tbsp
Orange (large), juice and grated rind	1	1
Egg (large)	1	1
Safflower oil	225 ml	8 fl oz
Skimmed milk	50–100 ml	2–4 fl oz
Carrots, grated	225 g	8 oz
Sultanas	50 g	2 oz
Walnuts, chopped	50 g	2 oz

1. Preheat oven to 180°C/350°F/Gas Mark 4. Oil and flour an 20-cm/8-in square cake tin.
2. Sift flours and baking powder into a bowl. Add fructose and ground almonds. Mix well.
3. Whisk orange juice, egg, oil and 50 ml/2 fl oz of skimmed milk. Pour liquid ingredients onto dry ingredients and mix well.
4. Stir in grated carrots, sultanas and walnuts. If mixture is too stiff, add remaining 50 ml/2 fl oz of skimmed milk.
5. Spoon mixture into prepared tin and bake for approximately 1 hour.

Makes 16 servings. 10 mg sodium approx. per serving.

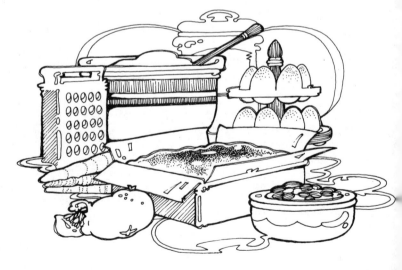

Apple and Raspberry Wholemeal Bread Pudding

	Metric	Imperial
Wholemeal bread, slightly stale medium thin slices, without crusts	6	6
Apples (Newtons or Granny Smiths)	750 g	1 ½ lb
Raspberries, fresh or frozen, no sugar added	500 g	1 lb
Zest and juice of lemon	1	1
Zest of juice of orange	1	1

Optional: sauce made with 225 g (8 oz) raspberries, puréed

1. Peel, core, quarter and slice apples. Place in a pan together with ¼ in. layer of water, lemon and orange juice and zest. Cover and simmer until apples are tender. Add raspberries and cook over a low heat for 5–10 minutes — until the juice of the raspberries just begins to run. Remove pan from heat and leave mixture until cold.

2. Line a 30 fl oz (1 ½ pt) pudding basin or soufflé with the bread slices cut to fit; spoon in the mixture plus the juices and top with remaining bread slices.

3. Cover uncooked pudding with plastic film then weight using a plate or saucer that fits inside the top of the pudding basin or soufflé dish and setting 2 lb kitchen weights or a similarly heavy weight like cans of food on top; refrigerate and leave overnight.

4. Use a flat-bladed knife to loosen edges and turn pudding out onto a serving dish. Spoon over any fruit juices that remain in the dish and serve with low fat yoghurt and extra purée if liked.

Serves 6. 15 mg sodium without the yoghurt

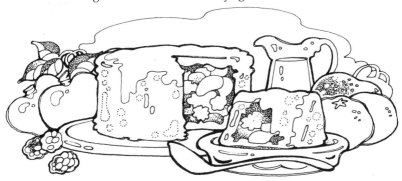

Appendix D

Addresses of PMS Clinics

The adequate treatment of PMS is very time consuming. Your own physician may prefer to refer you to a clinic which specializes in the care of PMS. This list of such clinics is as comprehensive and up-to-date as possible.

London
Elizabeth Garratt Anderson Hospital
PMS Clinic, Department of Gynaecology
Euston Road
LONDON NW1
Tel: 01–387 2501

PMS Clinic (Dr. K. Dalton)
100 Harley Street
LONDON W1
Tel: 01–935 2146

Marie Stopes Clinic
108 Whitfield Street
LONDON W1
Tel: 01–388 2585

St. George's Hospital
PMS Clinic, Department of Gynaecology
Tooting
LONDON SW17
Tel: 01–627 1255

St. Thomas's Hospital
PMS Clinic
St. Thomas's Hospital Medical School
LONDON SE1
Tel: 01–928 9292

University College Hospital (Dr. K. Dalton)
PMS Clinic
Gower Street
LONDON WC1

Women's Health Concern
17 Earl's Terrace
LONDON W8
01–602 6669

Out of London
Leeds General Infirmary
PMS Clinic
St. George Street
LEEDS
Tel: 0532–432799

Manchester Park Clinic
Wythenshawe
MANCHESTER
Tel: 061–437 2228

Sheffield Middleward Hospital
P.O. Box 134
SHEFFIELD
Tel: 0742–349491

National Association for Premenstrual Syndrome (NAPS)
PO Box 72
SEVENOAKS, Kent
Tel: 0732–459378
Helpline 0227–76133

Australia
Most of the teaching hospitals in Adelaide, Perth and Sydney
have PMS clinics associated. There is also:
The Samaritans (Australia)
60 Bagot road
Subiaco
PERTH W.A. 6008

Scotland
PMS Clinic
Stobhill Hospital
GLASGOW
Tel: 041–558 0111

PMS Clinic (Dr. Marion Hall)
Royal Infirmary
Foresterhill
ABERDEEN

Wales
PMS Clinic
Whitchurch Hospital
CARDIFF
Tel: 0222-62191

Appendix E

REHEARSING FOR THE NEW YOU

There are few things in life which provide the fun, health and sense of well-being exercise does. Jogging, tennis, swimming, cycling are all activities that, if done regularly, can help achieve your weight loss goal more quickly. In addition, a daily workout can help you look better, feel better and improve your posture and your self-confidence.

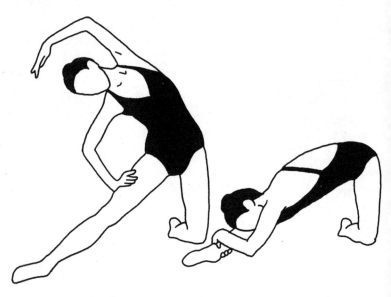

1 ALL OVER STRETCH

Firms up the midriff and stretches the leg muscles. Kneel with the right leg stretched straight out to the side. Place the right hand on the right leg, raise your left hand high over your head, bend to the right. Next, turn your upper body to face your right leg and reach, with both hands, as far down your leg as possible. Stretch very slowly, avoiding any jerky movements. Repeat on the other side. Start with 4 on each side and hold for 5 seconds. Each day, try to hold your leg farther down and gradually increase the holding time to 10 seconds.

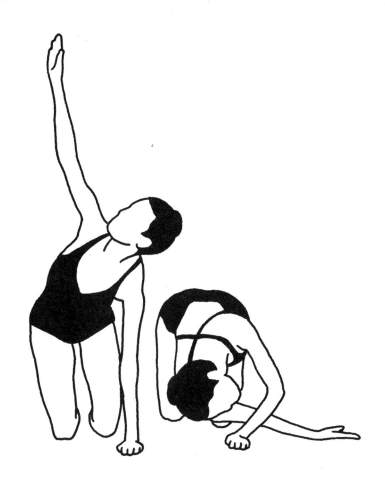

2   ARM FLING

An all-round upper body toner. Kneel on all fours. Curl the right arm under the left, touching the right shoulder to the floor. Slowly pull the right arm back out, and stretch it outwards and upwards toward the ceiling. Repeat with the other arm. Do 3 sets of 6 flings with each arm daily and increase to 4 sets of 10.

Note: this exercise routine was prepared with the cooperation of Canada's prima ballerina, Karen Kain.

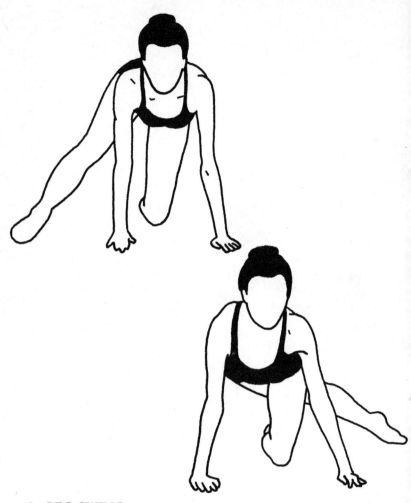

3 LEG SWING

Firms up hips and thighs. Kneel on all fours. Straighten one leg and swing this leg as far forward and to the side as possible, touching the floor. Return it gently and stretch it as far as possible in the opposite direction. Repeat using the other leg. Do 2 sets of 10 each on each leg (20 in all), and daily increase the number until you are doing 2 sets of 20, then 4 sets of 20. To make this one harder, try keeping the straight leg lifted off the floor, at shoulder height.

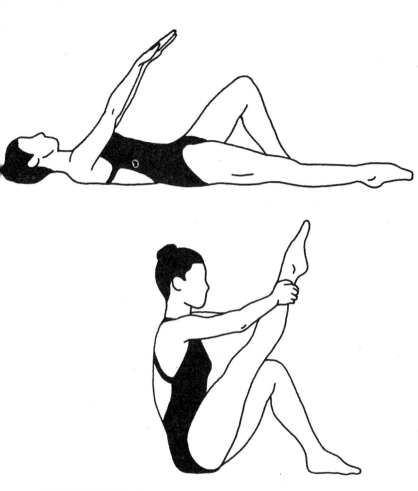

4 HALF JACKKNIFE

Strengthens stomach muscles & lower back. Lie on your back,
arms overhead, with one leg stretched out straight and the
other bent. Assume the pelvic tilt (as in exercise no. 5).
Slowly curl your upper body off the floor, bringing the arms
forward and lifting the straight leg. Grasp the straight leg and
gently pull it towards the body. Roll back to the starting
position and repeat with the other leg. Try 2 sets of 3
jackknives on each leg to begin with and gradually increase it
to 2 sets of 10.

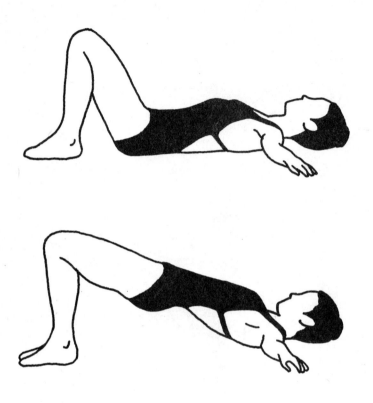

5 HIP LIFTS

Helps tighten the buttocks and back of thighs. Lie on your back
with the knees bent and your feet tucked about 6–10 inches
(15–25 cm) from your bottom. Rotate the pelvis and push the
lower back into the floor. This is called a pelvic tilt. Keeping
the tilt, raise buttocks off the floor until your body is in a
straight line from the shoulders to the knees. Do *not* arch
your back. Squeeze the buttocks and tense the abdominal
muscles on each lift. Slowly lower yourself back onto the
floor. Start with 10 hip lifts, holding them for 5 seconds each
and gradually increase to 20 daily.

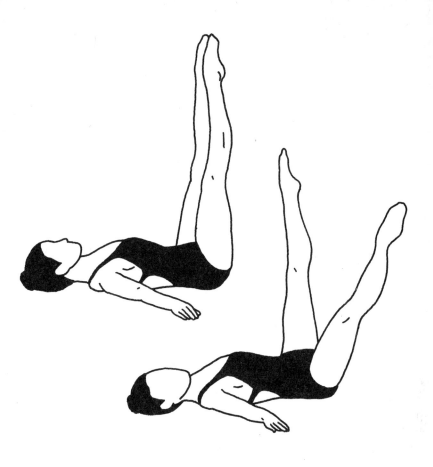

6 LEG SPLITS

Tones up inner thighs & lower stomach muscles. Lie on your back, with the arms stretched out at the sides at shoulder height and the knees bent. Tuck the knees to the chest, then straighten them towards the ceiling. (Don't let them drop back onto the floor while they are straight or you could strain your lower back). Keeping your shoulders and arms flat on the floor and your hips straight, slowly drop one leg out to the side as far as possible, then return it to a vertical position. Repeat with the other leg. Do 3 sets of 6 extensions on each leg at first, then gradually increase to 4 sets of 10. Remember to keep breathing evenly during this exercise.

Select Bibliography

Chapter 1 PMS: An Introduction

Dalton, K. (1982) "Legal Implications of PMS." *World Medicine* (17 April).

Dalton, K. and Laurence Taylor. (1983) "Pre-Menstrual Syndrome: A new criminal defence?" *California West Law Review* 19, no. 2.

Erickson, C. (1978) *Bloody Mary*. Garden City, New York: Doubleday.

Evans, W.A. (1932) *Mrs. Abraham Lincoln: A study of her personality and her influence on Lincoln*. New York: Knopf.

Frank, R.T. (1931) "Hormonal Causes of Pre-Menstrual Tension." *Archives of Neurology and Psychiatry* 26.

Plowden, A. (1972) *Marriage with my Kingdom*. New York: Stein & Day.

Regina v. Craddock. Current Law sect. 49, English Central Criminal Court (1981).

Regina v. English. Norwich Crown Court (10 November 1981).

Stassinopoulos, A. (1982) *Maria Callas*. New York: Ballantine Books.

Tingsten, H. (1972) *Victoria and the Victorians*. New York: Delacorte.

Chapter 2 Basics First: Inside Your Cycle

Dixon, H.G. (1982) *Undergraduate Obstetrics and Gynaecology*. Bristol: Wright.

Fuchs, F. (1982) "Behaviour and the Menstrual Cycle" in *An Overview — Pre-Menstrual Tension*. Edited by R. Friedman. New York: Marcel Dekker.

Gray's Anatomy. (1976) Edited by W.H. Lewis, Philadelphia: Lea and Febiger.

Johnson, M., and B. Everett. (1980) *Essential Reproduction*. Oxford: Blackwell.

Chapter 3 PMS: Symptoms and Causes

Abramovitz, E.S., and A.H. Baker. (1982) *American Journal of Psychiatry* 139, no. 4.

Bäckström, T. (1983) *Progesterone and Progestins*. Edited by C.W. Bardin et al. New York: Raven Press.

Brush, M.B., and D.F. Horrobin. (1983) International Symposium on Pre-Menstrual Tension and Dysmenorrhoea, South Carolina, USA.

Burke, L., and K. Gardner. (1982) *Why Suffer? Periods and their problems*. Second edition. London: Virago.

Collins-Williams, C. (1983) "The Atopic Patient." *Profiles in Practice* 2.

Dalton, K. (1959) "Menstruation and acute psychiatric illness." *British Medical Journal* 1, no.2.

Dalton, K. (1964) "Sickness, Menstruation, Time Lost at Work." *Proceedings Royal Society of Medicine* 57, no.4.

Dennerstein, L., and C. Spencer-Gardner. (1984) "Pre-Menstrual Tension: Hormonal Profiles." *Journal of Psychosomatic Obstetrics and Gynecology 3*, no.1.

Gray, L.A. (1941) *British Medical Journal* 3, no.34.

Greene, R., and K. Dalton. (1953) "The Premenstrual Syndrome." *British Medical Journal* 1.

Hart, R.D. (1960) *British Medical Journal* 1.

Holborow, J., and M. Lessof. (1983) "Immune Mechanisms in Health and Disease." *Medicine North America* 4.

Horrobin, D.F. (1973) *Prolactin, Physiology and Clinical Significance*. Lancaster: M.T.P. Press.

Horrobin, D.F. (1983) "The Role of Essential Fatty Acids and Prostaglandins in the Pre-Menstrual Syndrome." *Journal of Reproductive Medicine* 28.

Israel, S.L. (1938) *Journal of the American Medical Association* 110.

McCarron, D., and D. Henry. (1985) "Diet and Hypertension: Recent research." Cardiovascular Disease — Master Series, *Modern Medicine of Canada* 40, no. 8.

Merryman, W., et al. (1954) *Journal of Clinical Endocrinology* 14.

O'Brien, P., and E.M. Symonds. (1982) "Prolactin Levels in the Pre-Menstrual Syndrome." *British Journal of Obstetrics & Gynaecology* 89.

Reid, R., and S. Yen. (1981) "Pre-Menstrual Syndrome." *American Journal of Obstetrics and Gynecology* 139.

Richard, D., et al. (1971) "Pre-Menstrual Symptoms in self-referrals to a suicide prevention service." *British Journal of Psychiatry* 119.

Rothchild, I. (1983) *Progesterone and Progestins*. Edited by C.W. Bardin et al. New York: Raven Press

Siiteri, P.K. (1979) "Is Progesterone Nature's Immunosuppressant?" *Annals of New York Academy of Science* 286.

Smith, S., and C. Sauder. (1969) "Food cravings, depression and pre-menstrual problems." *Psychosomatic Medicine* 31, no.4.

Speroff, L., et al. (1983) *Clinical Endocrinology and Infertility*. London: Williams and Wilkins.

Speroff, L., and R. Van Weile. (1971) "Regulation of the Human Menstrual Cycle." *American Journal of Obstetrics and Gynecology* 109, no.2.

Wright, S., and J.L. Burton. (1982) "Oral Evening Primrose Oil Improves Atopic Eczema." *The Lancet* 2.

Chapter 4 Making the Diagnosis

Burke, L and K. Gardner. (1982) *Why Suffer? Periods and their problems*. Second edition. London: Virago.

Coppen, A., and N. Kessel. (1963) "Menstruation and Personality." *British Journal of Psychiatry* 109.

Dalton, K. (1968) "Menstruation and Examinations." *The Lancet* 11.

Ehrenreich, B., and D. English. (1973) *Complaints and Disorders: The Sexual Politics of Sickness*. Old Westbury, New York: The Feminist Press.

Moore, B. (1966) *I Am Mary Dunne*. New York: Viking.

Moos, R.H. (1968) "The development of a menstrual distress questionnaire." *Psychosomatic Medicine* 30.

Ruble, D.N. (1977) "Pre-Menstrual Symptoms: A Reinterpretation." *Science*.

Sanders, L. (1982) *The Third Deadly Sin*. New York: Berkley Books.

Schreeve, C. (1983) *PMS: The Curse that can be cured*. Wellingborough, England: Thorsons.

Chapter 5 The Treatment of PMS, Part I

Abraham, B. (1983) "Nutritional factors in the etiology of the Pre-Menstrual Tension Syndrome." *Journal of Reproductive Medicine* 28.

Abrahams, G.E., and J. Hargrove. (1980) "Effect of Vitamin B_6 on Pre-Menstrual Symptomatology in Women with PMS." *Infertility* 3.

Benson, H. (1975) *The Relaxation Response*. New York: Avon Books.

Brody, J. (1982) *Jane Brody's Nutrition Book*. New York: Bantam Books.

Budzynski, T., C.F. Stroebel and M.S. Schwartz. Three progressive relaxation tapes (audio-visual). New York: Guilford Publishing.

Burkitt, D.P. (1982) "Western diseases and their emergence related to diet." *South African Medical Journal* 61.

Chanarin, I. (n.d.) *The Megaloblastic Anaemias*. Oxford: Blackwell.

Chu, L., S. Yeh and D. Wood. (1979) *Acupuncture Manual: A Western approach*. New York: Marcel Dekker.

Cummings, J.H. (1981) "Dietary Fibre." *British Medical Bulletin* 37.

Dalton, K. (1982) "Behaviour and the Menstrual Cycle" in *An Overview — Pre-Menstrual Tension*. Edited by R. Friedman. New York: Marcel Dekker.

Fenly, L. (1984) "Dance-exercise guidelines planned." *Physician and Sportsmed* 9.

Friedman, M., and R.H. Rosenman. (1974) *Type A Behavior*. New York: Knopf.

Greenly, S., and H.H. Sandstead. (1980) "Zinc in human nutrition." *Modern Medicine of Canada* 35, no.10.

Growdon, J.H. and R.J. Wurtzman. (1980) "Nutrients and neurotransmitters." *Modern Medicine of Canada* 35, no.4.

Guillebaud, J. (1980) *The Pill*. Oxford: The Oxford University Press.

Holmes, T., and R. Rahe. (1967) "The Social Readjustment Rating Scale." *Journal of Psychosomatic Research* 11.

Horrobin, D.F. (1983) *Clinical Uses of Essential Fatty Acids*. Montreal: Eden Press.

Howard, J., D. Cunningham and P. Rechnitzer. (1978) *Rusting Out, Burning Out and Bowing Out*. Toronto: Macmillan.

Institute of Food Technologies. (1983) *Scientific Status Summary on Caffeine*. New York City: Valley Advocate Press.

Jencks, B. (1973) *Exercise Manual for J.H. Schultz's SAT and Special Formulas*. Salt Lake City: American Society of Clinical Hypnosis.

Lutter, J.M. (1983) "Mixed messages about osteoporosis in female athletes." *Physician and Sportsmed* 2, no.9.

McCance, R.A., and E.C. Widdowson. (1978) *The Composition of Foods*. Fourth edition. London: Her Majesty's Stationery Office.

McCarron, D., and D. Henry. (1985) "Diet and Hypertension: Recent research." Cardiovascular Disease Master Series, *Modern Medicine of Canada* 40, no.8.

O'Brien, P. (1980) *British Medical Journal* 1.

O'Brien, P., D. Craven and C. Selby. (1979) "Treatment of PMS by Spironalactone." *British Journal of Obstetrics & Gynaecology* 86.

Pelletier, K.R. (1977) *Mind as Healer, Mind as Slayer: A Holistic approach to preventing stress disorders*. New York: Delacorte.

Pfeiffer, C. (1975) "Mental and Elemental Nutrients."
    Physicians Desk Reference.
Prior, J.C. (1985) "Hormonal mechanisms of reproductive
    function, and hypothalamic adaptation to endurance
    training." *Human Kinetics.*
Selye, H. (1974) *Stress Without Distress.* Philadelphia:
    Lippincott.
Shephard, R.J. (1982) "Prognostic value of exercise testing."
    British Journal of Sports Medicine 16.
Spiller, G.A. (1976) *Fibre in Human Nutrition.* New York and
    London: Plenum Press.
Stamford, B. (1984) "Aerobic dance: good for fitness."
    Physician and Sportsmed 4.
Streiff, R. (1970) "Folate deficiency and oral contraceptives."
    Journal of the American Medical Association 214.
Thornton, Ward B. (1978) "Folic acid, mental functions and
    dietary habits." *Journal of Clinical Psychiatry* 39.
Watts, G. (1982) "Linoleic Acid in Medicine." *World Medicine*
    (January).
Wilson, R.C.D. (1983) "Cardiovascular Disease: Prevention in
    Practice." *British Columbia Medical Journal* 25, no.9.

Chapter 5 The Treatment of PMS, Part II

Andersch, B. (1983) "Bromocryptine and pre-menstrual
    symptoms: Survey of double-blind trials." *Obstetrics &
    Gynaecology Survey* 38.
Nilluis, S.J., and E.D.B. Johansson. (1971) "Plasma levels after
    Progesterone Suppository Therapy." *American Journal of
    Obstetrics and Gynecology* 110, no.40.
Nilluis, S.J., and E.D.B. Johansson. (1971) "Progesterone
    Suppository Therapy: Comparative Rectal and Vaginal
    Routes." *Acta Endocrinologica* 1.
Van Der Meer, Y., et al. (1983) "Effects of high-dose
    progesterone on PMS." *Journal of Psychosomatic Obstetrics and
    Gynecology* 2.

Chapter 6 Additional Factors Affecting PMS

Barnes, L.A., and Y.A. Cable. (1981) *Nutrition and Medical
    Practice.* Connecticut: Avi Publishing.
Canada. Department of National Health and Welfare. (1984)
    "Food additives: Questions and Answers."
Crook, W. (1986) *The Yeast Connection.* New York: Random
    House.

Feingold, B.F. (1975) *Why Your Child is Hyperactive*. New York: Random House.

Freydberg, N., and W.A. Sortner. (1982) *The Food Additives Book*. London and Toronto: Bantam Books.

Grant, E.C. (1979) "Food Allergy and Migraine." *The Lancet* 1.

Haddad, Z.H. (1982) "Clinical and immunological aspects of food hypersensitivity." (Bela Schick Memorial Lecture.) *Annals of Allergy* 49.

Hodges, R.E. (1980) *Nutrition in Medical Practice*. London: W.B. Saunders.

International Task Force Expert Panel on Food Safety and Nutrition. (1972) "Nitrites, and Nitrosamines in Foods: A Dilemma." *Journal of Food Sciences* 37.

Jones, V.A., et al. (1982) "Food intolerance: A Major factor in the pathogenesis of irritable bowel syndrome." *The Lancet* 2.

King, D.S., and M. Mandell. (1981) "Can allergic exposure provoke psychological symptoms?" *Biological Psychology* 26.

Patel, D.G., and W.G. Thompson. (1985) "Gluten in Pills: A hazard for patients with celiac disease." *Canadian Medical Association Journal* 133.

Rowe, A.H. (1972) *Food Allergy. Its manifestations and control, and the elimination diets: A Compendium*. Springfield, Ill.: C.C. Thomas.

Truss, O.C. (1983) *The Missing Diagnosis*. Birmingham, Ala.: O.C. Truss.

Winter, R. (1978) *Consumer's Dictionary of FoodAdditives*. New York: Craven Publishing.

Recipe and Diet Index

General Index

additives, 75–80
adrenalin, 26
aerobics, 62
alcohol, 54
allergies, 27, 73–5
amines, 28, 46, 65
amino acids, 47–8
angiotensin, II, 19
anorexia, 61
anti-depressants, 65–6
antioxidants, 78–9
ascorbic acid, 52
asthma, 38

bananas, 46
B-complex vitamins, 50–1
blood sugar levels, 19, 26, 45, 48
bran, 47
breast discharge, 38
breast milk, 26
bromocriptine, 66
bulimia, 61

caffeine, 42–3
calcium, 52–4
calisthenics, 61–2
Candida albicans, 70–3
candidiasis, 68
carbohydrates, 26, 45, 48
cervical dysplasia, 52
coeliac disease, 74
colouring agents, 76–7, 78
conception, 15
contraceptives, oral, 10, 52, 54–5
corpus luteum, 13, 15
cramps, 17, 19, 23

daily food-monitoring chart, 34
Dalton, Katharina, 11
Danazol, 66–7
delta-6-desaturase, 49
depression, 38, 46, 65–6
diuretics, 65
doctors, 29–30
dolomite, 54

dopamine, 23, 66
dydrogesterone, 67

Efamol, 49
emulsifiers, 79
endometriosis, 67
endometrium, 13, 15, 17
endorphins, 22
essential fatty acids, 23–4
exercise, 61–2

fats, 48 *see also* essential fatty
acids
fibre, 46–7
flavouring aids, 44
folic acid, 52
Frank, Robert T., 11
fruit, 48
FSH (follicle stimulating
hormone), 12, 17

gamma-linolenic acid (GLA),
24–6, 48–50
gluten, 74
gonadotrophins, 12
Greene, Raymond, 11

headaches, 23, 38, 46
hormones, 9, 10, 12, 17
HPO (hypothalamus-pituitary-
ovary) nerve linkup, 21–2, 23
hypoglycaemia, 19, 26–7
hypothalamus, 10, 12, 15, 17, 23,
66

immune system, 27, 73
immunoglobins, 27
insulin, 26

key regime, 42
for severe PMS, 63–4

Lactobacillus acidophilus, 71–2
libido, 21
linoleic acid, 24–6, 48–50

121

Notes